YOUR WOUNDS I WILL HEAL

PRAYER FOR INNER HEALING

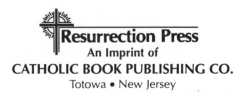

Robert Faricy, SJ
Lucy Rooney, SND deN
Foreword by George Maloney, SJ

Resurrection Press
An Imprint of
CATHOLIC BOOK PUBLISHING CO.
Totowa • New Jersey

First published as "Praying for Inner Healing" by Robert Faricy, SJ in 1979 by Paulist Press.

Published in August, 1999 by Resurrection Press, Ltd.
P.O. Box 248
Williston Park, NY 11596

ISBN 1-878718-53-3

Library of Congress Catalog Card Number 99-70151

Cover design by John Murello

Printed in Canada.

1 2 3 4 5 6 7 8 9

"Your hurt is incurable;
your wound cannot be healed.
There is no one to cure you,
no medicine to make you well,
no healing for you.

Why do you complain about your hurt?
Your pain is incurable.

But I will restore you to health,
and your wounds I will heal,"
says the Lord.

JER 30:12-13, 15, 17

This book is for Beth Benepe.

Contents

Foreword by George Maloney, S.J.   7

Introduction   9

Part I INNER HEALING

    Chapter 1   Praying to be Healed   13

    Chapter 2   The Truth of Myself and
                  the Mercy of the Lord   35

    Chapter 3   Crying Out to the Lord   45

Part II THE CROSS AND INNER HEALING

    Chapter 4   By His Wounds We are Healed   63

    Chapter 5   The Cross and Prayer
                  for Inner Healing   77

    Chapter 6   Jesus' Mother at the Cross   91

Part III JESUS, THE GIFTS OF THE SPIRIT
AND INNER HEALING

Chapter 7 Being Healed through Praise
and the Gifts of the Spirit   101

Chapter 8 Jesus Is Lord   115

Chapter 9 A Prayer for Inner Healing   129

Notes   139

Foreword

THERE IS NOT ONE WHO READS THESE WORDS who cannot claim his or her share of brokenness. This shows itself at various times of our lives in varying degrees of intensity. We can all see the progressive degrees of physical brokenness as we move each day a bit closer to that final earthly moment of total dissolution from our material existence.

But what brokenness we find in our psychic order! What fears assail us with unceasing cruelty day and night! Doubts, anger, depression, hatred and unforgiveness seethe within us as a gigantic, smoldering volcano that needs the slightest tremor to pour forth its molten lava in cruel actions, biting words or fitful retreat into lonely solitude.

Then there are the terrifying dark nights of the spiritual world. We cry out to see again the face of God. Yet there is only darkness! Not only does God seem to be absent, but we seem to have lost all faith in him. What blasphemous thoughts possess us! Down deeper I am forced to go into my life. How do I know God really exists? That Jesus is really the Son of God and will come to our help?

In all of this we cringe in our brokenness, hoping, begging, searching for a way out of such absurdity and utter meaninglessness. Does God truly love me? Can he answer my prayers and bring me into a new creation?

A Healing Savior

For true Christians, Jesus Christ is the Way that heals the world of its brokenness. He has come among us in order to bring us life, that we might have it more abundantly (Jn 10:10). He has inserted himself as the Divine Word into our broken, human condition in order that he might become one like us in all things save sin (Heb 4: 25). More than becoming one like us, he remains always the Image of the heavenly Father (Col 1:15), one with him in his Spirit of love.

It is this loving Spirit that gives us an experience of God the Father's infinite love for us individually, made manifest to us by Jesus. As in his lifetime on this earth, so now, Jesus, the risen Lord, is filled with love and compassion for all of us not yet freed from our enslavement to sin and death. We must first believe that he is still alive and living in his members, the Church. Through the Church we can truly encounter the risen Lord and our Savior in the preached Good News and in the sacraments. We must give our lives entirely to him by placing him at the center of all our desires and values instead of our self-centered selves.

We must forgive others and keep his commandments, especially that of loving one another as he loves us. As we grow into greater wholeness, Christ will work through us also to bring healing to those human beings whom we encounter in the concrete human situations of every day.

I heartily recommend this latest book by Father Robert Faricy, S.J. and Sister Lucy Rooney, SNDdeN. *Your Wounds I Will Heal: Praying for Inner Healing* was first published as *Praying for Inner Healing* by Paulist Press twenty years ago. This new edition is a revision and expansion of the earlier edition and I have been struck by the richness the co-authors have brought to this new edition.

The authors present here an excellent and quite complete work on Christian healing, starting with an overview and exegesis of relevant passages of the Old and New Testament. What struck me in this new edition is the stress placed on prayer, both on the part of those in the healing ministry and for all persons seeking healings.

Much modern psychology has been used by the authors in order to give practical ways of praying for healings that complement Christian and also psychological teachings, as Vatican II Council stressed in its *Pastoral Constitution on the Church in the Modern World*. This book will bring enlightenment and great encouragement to all seeking healings from the Triune God and knowledge and motivation to those already involved in the healing ministry to bring health and greater life into the Body of Christ.

GEORGE A. MALONEY, S.J.

Introduction

FIRST, A NOTE TO THE READER. This book is a revision and an expansion of *Praying for Inner Healing* written eighteen years ago to help each of us to pray for our own inner healing. It contains many references to scripture and much theology; we try to present food for reflection and for prayer, not at all watered down, but presented in such a way as to be practical.

> *"Out of his infinite glory*
> *may he give you the power through*
> *his Spirit for your inner self to grow strong."*
>
> EPH 3:16

That quest for our inner self and its healing, has brought many people to ask for prayer for healing so that they may live more joyfully and serve the Lord more effectively. So, with the co-operation of Emile Cerar of Resurrection Press, we have decided to update and expand *Praying for Inner Healing* because we think that the Lord will work through it, still, in these days, so that his desire might be fulfilled, that:

> *"we might exist for the praise of his glory."*
>
> EPH 1:12

> *"with a diadem instead of ashes,*
> *the oil of gladness instead of mourning,*
> *a glorious mantle instead of a downcast spirit."*
>
> IS 61:3

9

Does prayer for inner healing really work? Is it powerful? Yes. It works, powerfully. Not because prayer is powerful, but because the Lord loves each of us — you and me — and because his love has power to heal us. If you ask him for a piece of bread, he will not give you a stone. If you ask him for inner healing, do you really think he will do nothing?

Why does the Lord listen to you, answer your prayers, heal you when you ask him to? Because he knows your name, he calls you by your name, he knows your heart through and through, and he loves you. He loves you unconditionally, without any qualification, with no reservations. He does not say, "Let me heal you, and then I will love you more." He does not say, "Shape up, and then I will love you more." He does not shake his finger at you. He loves you maximally, now. And he will do anything that you ask, to help you.

Praying for inner healing is not a technique, not in any way a skill or a set of tricks. It is not psychology. It is prayer.

Praying for inner healing, like all prayer, is just the opposite of technique. Magic is technique, spiritual technology. Magic tries to manipulate God, to somehow force him to do what I want him to do. Magic does not work on God. He will not be manipulated.

What works is turning to the Lord in childlike humility. He loves us and he cannot resist us.

We look for the right book, for the right technique, for the best method, for some kind of spiritual technology, some course we could follow. And all the time, Jesus is there. Here, really. Ready and wanting to help. It is enough to turn to him, to cry out to him, to ask him to heal me.

How do I pray for inner healing? Any way I can. And remembering that it is the Lord who does the healing, not me, not my prayer.

We want to thank all those who have taught us about praying for inner healing, and particularly Sister Margaret Tracey, Eileen Kennedy, Diana Villegas, Francis McNutt, Dennis Hamm, and Matthew and Dennis Linn.

Lucy Rooney, SND de N
Robert Faricy, SJ

London and Rome
Pentecost 1998

Part I

INNER HEALING

❧

ONE

Praying to be Healed

IN RECENT YEARS, the interest in healing as a response to prayer has grown greatly. Besides the traditional Christian faith in the power of prayer, other factors contribute to this growth of interest: in particular, the charismatic renewal, in which healings of different kinds occur frequently, and the renewal of the sacraments of healing, i.e. the sacraments of Reconciliation, of the Anointing of the Sick, and of the Eucharist. This chapter outlines briefly the basis, in scripture and in Christian practice, of prayer for healing, and it describes prayer for healing, especially prayer for inner healing.

Healing in the New Testament

In the gospels, healings take up twenty per cent (in Luke's gospel, one third) of the text. Jesus' ministry is not only to teach, but also to heal; in fact, his self-concept includes, integrally, the idea of being a healer. In the synagogue at Nazareth he applies Isaiah 61:1,2 to himself:

"The Spirit of the Lord is upon me.
He has anointed me to bring good news to the poor.
He has sent me to give liberty to the captives
and sight to the blind,
And to set free the oppressed."

LK 4:18

When John's disciples come to ask him who he is, they find him curing "many of diseases and plagues and evil spirits," and giving sight to many blind people. He answers them:

"Tell John what you have seen and heard: the blind
receive their sight, the lame walk, the lepers are
cleansed, the deaf hear, the dead are raised,
the poor have good news preached to them."

LK 7:22

Jesus' healings are signs of the times, signs of the presence of the Kingdom of God in him. The Kingdom-to-come is already present in the public ministry of Jesus. This is clear from the fact that Jesus acts in the power of the Spirit, the Spirit of the "last times," when God will pour out his Spirit in the coming of his Kingdom.

"I will pour out my Spirit on all flesh:
your sons and your daughters shall prophesy,
your old people shall dream dreams,
and your young people shall see visions.
Even on male and female slaves,
in those days I will pour out my Spirit."

JOEL 2:28-29

In the past, perhaps we have not always understood the healings in the gospel in the way that they are presented for our understanding. Jesus' healings have been seen chiefly as demonstrations, even proofs, of his divinity or of his messianic authenticity. In the gospels, however, the "miracle" aspect, although there, is not accentuated. What is underlined, rather, is that God had come to save us. The power of God is present in Jesus to heal us, to save us. The healings that Jesus works are part of, and reveal, the divine work of our salvation.

Not all the gospel cures are physical. Some are spiritual healings: Jesus forgives sins and counsels the sinners to change their lives. And some seem to be psychological healings. Among Jesus' many exorcisms, in which the power of the Spirit of Jesus is contrasted with and seen in opposition to every spirit opposed to God, there appear to be some that are emotional or psychological cures rather than true exorcisms. In the time of the formation of the gospels, mental illness had not yet been seen as a category of human behavior; it would have been normal to associate psychoses and grave neuroses with the forces of evil, attributing them to unclean or evil spirits. It seems likely that some of the healings that were understood as exorcisms were in reality psychological healings.

All Jesus' healings are the fruit of his compassion. This compassion, the most obvious quality of his personality (today as then), and the motivation for his healing ministry, is strongly present in his teaching. He not only forgives sinners — the woman taken in adultery, the paralytic on his mat, Peter, and others — but he also teaches forgiveness. In particular, he preaches the compassion of God for sinners; several parables have divine compassion as their central point. The God of Jesus' parables is a God who searches out those who need him and his forgiveness: the shepherd searches for the lost sheep; the housewife lights a lamp and sweeps out her house, looking for a lost coin; and the father stands out on the road looking for his son, and finally sees him even while still a long way off. The parable of the prodigal son is not so much about the son as about the prodigal father, prodigal with compassion, forgiveness and goodness. What kind of a person would invent such parables? A person whose own compassion and love was so great that, on his entrance into Jerusalem, ordinary people took off their coats and threw them before him to make a carpet in the street, cut branches off the trees, waved them and threw them too, and acted so exuberantly as to incur the censure of the leaders of Israel. Jesus is the revelation of the Father; the Father's compassion is mirrored in all Jesus' relationships with others. His table ministry to the prostitutes and tax collectors, especially, shows his compassion. When criticized for his conduct, Jesus replies:

> *"Those who are well have no need of the doctor,*
> *but those who are sick;*
> *I came to call not the righteous, but sinners."*
>
> MK 2:17

Breaking bread with sinners is part of his healing ministry; he sees himself as a doctor, a healer.

Jesus' compassionate love has an unrelenting and uncompromising force. Certain parables reflect this 'all-out' aspect of his mercy and love. In the teaching that the Kingdom of Heaven is like a treasure hidden in a field that one buys after selling all other possessions, or like a pearl of great price that a merchant sells all his other pearls to buy, we find Jesus' own attitude towards the Kingdom. He has come to plant the Kingdom in each of us; *the Kingdom of God is within you* (Lk 17:21), so that in a sense, each of us is the Kingdom for him. That is, each person, for Jesus, is the treasure hidden in the field that, giving up everything else, he buys. And each of us is the pearl of great price; *you have been ransomed . . . with the precious blood of Christ* (1 Pet 1:19).

Jesus' disciples continue his ministry of healing (Lk 9: 1-2;9:11;10:8-9). Jesus is, we might say, "multiplied" in his disciples; his healing power works through them. In the Acts of the Apostles healing is an integral part of the church's ordinary ministry. In Jesus' name, Peter heals the man lame from birth at the gate called Beautiful (Acts 3: 6-7), and Paul heals the cripple at Lystra (Acts 14:10). People place the sick so that at least Peter's shadow can fall on them (Acts 5:15), and handkerchiefs and aprons that Paul had touched are brought to the sick — who are healed. Crowds came to Peter for healing (Acts 5:16), just as the Maltese are healed when they come to Paul. A wide variety of ills are healed, ranging from dysentery (Acts 28:8) to complete paralysis (Acts 9:34) and even death (Acts 9:40;20:10). Healings come about also through Stephen, Philip and Ananias of Damascus; but Peter and Paul are the most important. They stand for the church as a whole, and teach us that Jesus heals in and through his church.

Christian Healing Today[1]

According to the promises of Christ:

> *"These signs will accompany those who believe . . .*
> *they will lay their hands on the sick,*
> *who will recover."*

MK 16:17-18

> *"Truthfully, I tell you, the one who believes in me*
> *will also do the works that I do and, in fact, will do*
> *even greater works than these, because I am going*
> *to the Father."*

JN 14:12

Healings in response to prayer continue; today, they happen with extraordinary frequency, and they certainly constitute a sign of our times. Christian tradition, of course, has always included healings due to God's compassionate intervention. Down through the centuries saints have worked miraculous cures, and praying with faith for the sick has always been part of Christianity. And there have always been shrines at which miraculous cures take place, like Guadalupe, Lourdes and Fatima. Today, however, due to the charismatic renewal and to the renewal of the sacraments of healing, the healing power of the Spirit stands out perhaps more than at any time since early Christianity.

The sacrament of Reconciliation is the sacrament of spiritual healing. Spiritual healing consists in receiving God's forgiveness and, at the same time, his power to live in a more Christian way. This double grace, to be forgiven and to do better, is a healing of the soul. Sometimes, in the sacrament of Reconciliation, grace overflows and touches in a healing way not only the spiritual but the psychological roots of sinful tendencies; in such cases we can speak of psychological healing. Most confessors have experienced this kind of healing in penitents, healing at both the spiritual and the emotional levels. The renewal of this sacrament has stressed these healing aspects. This is not to be wondered at, for sin usually begins in the mind before it is acted out, so it is the mind which needs healing and forgiving. It is well, in preparing for this sacrament, to ask the Lord to heal the roots of the sins we intend to confess. We may be able to identify anger, pride, lack of love, or whatever *root of bitterness* (Heb 12:15) is at the heart of our sin. The power of the sacrament of Reconciliation should not be underestimated. It contains not only all the love God has for us, but the whole saving life and death of Jesus.

The renewal of the sacrament of the Anointing of the Sick too, has stressed the sacrament's healing power. This renewal has reoriented the purpose of the sacrament from a preparation for death to the complete healing, spiritual and psychological and physical, of all who are seriously sick. This is in keeping with the practice of the early church according to the Letter of James. In fact, the important text of James' letter is read early in the liturgy of the sacrament of the sick:

> *"Is any among you sick? Let him send for the elders of the church, and let them pray over him, anointing him with oil in the name of the Lord; and the prayer of faith will save the sick man, and the Lord will raise him up; and if he has sinned, he will be forgiven."*
>
> JAS 5:14-15

The Eucharist, too, must be considered as a sacrament of healing. After the Second Vatican Council, the renewal of the Mass resulted in a clearer understanding of the sacramental grace of the Eucharist: the formation of Christian community. This idea, traditional but rediscovered, includes the notion of the healing of interpersonal relationships.

> *"Because there is one bread, we although many are one body, for we all partake of the one bread."*
>
> 1 COR 10:17

We are one body of Christ, because we each receive the one body of Christ. The Eucharist is, at the same time, a sacrament of the healing of the individual person. The Mass is a celebration of healing — of body, mind and spirit — of the whole person, of our past and present, and a safeguard against future ills.

> *I eat your body and drink your blood. Let it . . .*
> *bring me health in mind and body.*
>
> PRAYER BEFORE COMMUNION

> *Lord, through this sacrament may we rejoice in*
> *your healing power and experience your saving*
> *love in mind and body.*
>
> 1st MONDAY OF LENT, POST COMMUNION

As the celebrant holds the host high, the congregation prays together: *Say but the word and I shall be healed.* After receiving Communion, we can ask the Lord within us to shine his healing light, or lay his hand on those areas where healing is needed.

The charismatic renewal, which had its beginnings in the Pentecostalism of the turn of the century, entered the mainline Protestant churches and the Roman Catholic church in the 1960s. This renewal has been a shower of graces and gifts and, particularly, of charisms. A charism is a special gift, given not to all but only to some, for the building up of the community. There are many charisms, including teaching, counselling, evangelizing, leading, prophecy, miracles and healing. The new outpouring of the charism of healing, sometimes on individuals and sometimes on groups, has resulted in large numbers of healings of many kinds.

Inner Healing

The most important kind of healing is spiritual healing. In fact, experience shows that physical healing received as

an answer to prayer invariably includes, and as a pre-
dominant element, a deeper conversion of heart, a new
adhesion to the Lord — that is, a spiritual healing. Of
course, the physical, the psychological and the spiritual
overlap, touch and influence one another; in practice, they
can be distinguished but not separated. Spiritual healing
will have a psychological component, and psychological
healing will often have a physical component in the form
of better physical health. Also, some physical ills have
their origins, at least partially, in emotional disorders; the
healing of emotional problems can sometimes radically
improve or even completely heal biological illness.

This section describes inner healing.[2] By the term "inner
healing" we mean both spiritual and psychological healing; our approach here will be along the lines of the psychological, but without neglecting the spiritual.

Ordinarily, prayer for inner healing does not take place
in a large group, although it can, but rather on a one-to-
one basis, or with perhaps two people praying for the
inner healing of a third. A confessor can pray for inner
healing for a penitent during or immediately after the
sacrament of Reconciliation. One can also pray alone for
one's own inner healing — and this is the most common.

What is prayer for inner healing? All of us, at least
sometimes, have experienced inner suffering, or conflicts,
or strong and unreasonable anger or fear or sadness. We
know from the gospels that Jesus can heal us, not only
physically, but also interiorly, psychologically, emotional-
ly, spiritually. We know, too, that prayers are answered.

Often the Lord will work through some people to heal
others, for example, through psychological counselling.
However, Jesus also heals simply in answer to prayer for
inner healing. This means that we can pray for and with
others that they may be healed in their emotions, and it

means that we ourselves can pray to be healed interiorly. Jesus said explicitly that he has come *to set captives free* (Lk 4:18). He does this by setting us free from the inner hurts which can warp our lives and are often the roots of sin. The things we have done, for which we feel shame or remorse; the words we regret saying, but cannot now take back, these are interior hurts we have inflicted on ourselves. Jesus loves us into forgiveness, but even more — to the healing of those wounds. Inner healing is always, ultimately a healing of relationships — even, and perhaps first, our relationship with self. The overt harm that others have done to us is more easily seen, and we will return to that.

We know from psychology and psychiatry that much of what needs to be healed in us is buried beneath the level of consciousness. Interior suffering or stress or sadness frequently results from root problems or hurts or wounds or conflicts that are not conscious, that we are not aware of. We see only the tips of the icebergs that need to be melted. It is not necessary to know with precision what needs healing, although it helps. We can pray to be healed, interiorly, in our emotions, insofar as we are aware that we need healing, and then we can let the Lord take it from there and guide us to what we should do or pray for next.

Where do these — mostly unconscious — hurts come from? They come from the very beginning of our existence, from our earliest years, from our childhood and growing up, from the whole process of living. Some of them are so early and so deeply repressed that we can never get at them; but Our Lord sees them all, with love, and can heal them all. Many interior wounds, both conscious and buried, result from poor or inadequate home life in childhood, from negative aspects of school life, from setbacks in childhood or in later life. In many cases, things have been done to people which ought never to have been done, a lot of suffering was caused, and healing is needed.

In general, and without making rigid classifications, we can distinguish three kinds of prayer for inner healing. We can pray for healing of the heart, of the affective drives; often the reasons for a negative state are unknown, or vague, or dispersed, but the affectivity seems disturbed in such a way that the resulting emotions tend to block progress in union with God. Examples are a relative incapacity to love or to receive the love of others, a timidity that severely limits communication with others, general depression. Such problems no doubt have their roots, at least partly, in buried memories, but often these memories are inaccessible. Sometimes, especially in the case of depressive personalities, looking for root memories can bring to the surface psychological conflicts that might better remain unconscious or that require the attention of a psychologist or psychiatrist. In asking others to pray with us for inner healing, we should be vigilant in ensuring that they are persons of discretion who will honor confidentiality. They should also be people of good sense, as well as being spiritual. Even professional psychiatrists can become ensnared in "false memory syndrome." *Discern everything* says Paul (1 Cor 2:15).

Secondly, we can pray for liberation from a habit or tendency that goes against progress in union with God. For example, we can pray that the Lord free us from excessive suspiciousness, or from selfishness, or from fear, or from patterns of undesirable behavior, or from depression.

Another way to pray for inner healing is to pray for healing of memories. We can simply ask the Lord to bring to mind any past memory or memories that he wants to heal. Then we can ask him to heal that memory. Memories to be healed might be childhood memories of an over-strict father or a possessive mother, or of an alcoholic or otherwise ill parent, or of poverty, or loneliness, or fear of a certain teacher, or shame at being too fat, or of being mocked as inadequate or handicapped, or suffering an accident or physical abuse, or a thousand other things. These trouble-causing memories will be found to contain one or more of the four typical reactions to stress: anger (or bitterness or resentment), fear (or withdrawal), anxiety, or guilt feelings.

In prayer, I can take the Lord's hand and let him walk back in time, in my own personal history, to the time and place where I was hurt. I can ask him to be present in that hurtful situation — in the home, or in the classroom, or on the playground — filling it with his healing love. And I ask him to take the pain out of the memory, to remove all fear and anxiety and guilt and anger associated with that memory, and to fill the places where they were, with his love. I pray not that the memory disappear, but that its meaning be changed so that I can praise God and even thank him for what happened, knowing that he writes straight with crooked lines and that the healed memory will mean the conversion of past hurts into greater understanding of the hurts of others, into a broader and deeper compassion, or into some other positive force. As people grow older they frequently have flashbacks to incidents, places, and persons of their past. These are moments for asking the Lord to be present in those episodes, happy or regretful, and to praise and thank him, or to ask him to put right anything which is troubling. If we are praying with a dying person, they may have things which still disturb them, "unfinished business." We can, if they wish, pray for inner healing. Or, they may just want, like John at the Last Supper, to lean on the Lord's heart, and trust him with everything, as their prayer becomes simple and undetailed.

The Conditions of Inner Healing

What do we need to do to dispose ourselves prayerfully to let the Lord heal us interiorly? What are the conditions of inner healing? There are three: faith — that we believe in Jesus' power to heal us personally; repentance; and for-giveness of others.

God acts in and through Jesus. And he asks us to believe not only in his love but also in his power, for his love is powerful and it heals. Believing in Jesus' love for me is one thing; more is needed — to believe in the force of his love, in the healing power of his compassion for me personally. Jesus knows all my life, he remembers — he was there at my conception as he has been every moment since, calling me by name.

> "But now, says the Lord,
> he who created you . . .
> he who formed you in the womb . . .
> Do not fear, for I have redeemed you;
> I have called you by name,
> You are mine."
>
> IS 43:1

> "I have loved you with an everlasting love;
> therefore I have continued to be faithful to you."
>
> JER 31:3

> "With everlasting love I will have compassion on
> you, says the Lord your Redeemer."
>
> IS 54:8

Only a conviction (not necessarily a feeling) of the Lord's unique love for me as I am, can open me to his healing love so that he can free me from the chains of past and present hurts, to walk with him in his love, and to let it overflow. A crippled heart has no energy for others. The chains that bind us to Jesus are very different:

> *"I led them with cords of kindness,*
> *with leading strings of love.*
> *I was for them like one*
> *who lifts up an infant."*

HOS 11:4

The healing power of the humanity of Jesus is surely not less than it was when he helped people during his public ministry; if anything, it is greater after his resurrection. And he has promised us that he hears and answers our prayers.

The second condition of inner healing is repentance. This includes the renunciation of sin and a conversion, a turning towards God in humility to accept his mercy and forgiving love. But perhaps the very thing for which a person might seek healing is a chronic sin for which they are not fully sorry — otherwise they would be already on the way to healing. They may not be able, convincingly, to renounce the sin, but they can turn to God in humility, confessing the double healing they need. It helps to remember that the Lord came to save not the just, but sinners, and that my very sinfulness attracts his loving compassion, that the dark side of myself, that I find so hard to accept, he accepts totally and lovingly, and that my very weakness is the opening in me to him and to his saving strength which is made perfect in my weakness.

I want to accept the Lord's forgiveness and to let him heal me. This means encountering him in prayer in terms of the disorder in my life; it means coming before the mer-

ciful Lord as the sinful, hurt, disordered person that I am.
I want to be aware, in the light of the Lord's love, of my
sinfulness, of the dark side of myself, aware that I am held
captive in a sinful frame of reference so that he can minis-
ter to the effects of sin in me — original sin, my personal
sins, and the sins and imperfections of others. To do this,
I want to be centered not on myself and my sins, nor on
some experience that I want to have of the Lord, but on
the forgiving Lord himself, going to him, small, lowly, and
simply, like a child, knowing that the initiative is his, not
mine, knowing that he called me to be forgiven and
healed, before I ever thought of it myself.

The third condition of inner healing is that we forgive
others.

> *"Put on compassion, kindness, lowliness,*
> *gentleness, patience. Be forbearing with one*
> *another, and if one has a complaint against*
> *someone else, forgive one another. As the Lord has*
> *forgiven you, so too you also must forgive."*
>
> COL 3:12-13

This can be difficult. Or I can think I have adequately
forgiven someone, when in fact resentment still remains
in my heart.

Jesus tells me to come to him if I labor and am weighed
down; and he will give me rest. To open my heart to Jesus,
I have to forgive others. I need to forgive others so the
shell I have built around my heart, the shell of unforgiveness, the crust, the hardness, will go. And this, so that
Jesus can heal my heart of the hurts others have caused
me. To receive God's forgiving and healing love, I need to
forgive others.

After teaching his disciples the "Our Father," Jesus

adds this sentence by way of explanation and emphasis:

> *"Yes, if you do forgive others their sins and failings against you, then your Father in heaven will forgive you your sins and failings. But if you do not forgive others, then neither will your Father forgive you your sins and failings."*
>
> MT 6:14-15

Failure to forgive other persons the pain and the hurt that they have caused me can block me, can close me to the healing power of Jesus. The resentment or the anger that I feel towards a person who has hurt me can act as a hard shell around the inner wound that person caused. That hard casing of resentment or bitterness can screen the hurt from Jesus' healing power. If I hold another bound by unforgiveness, then my own heart and life are bound too:

> *"Whatever you bind on earth will be bound also in heaven."*
>
> MT 16:19

If I set the other free by forgiving, I am set free too. The poison has to stop somewhere or be continually passed on. Jesus, on the cross absorbed all sin and hatred into himself, and put an end to it:

> *"He forgave us all our sins, erasing the record that stood against us with its legal demands. He set the record aside, nailing it to the cross."*
>
> COL 2:14

But if an inability to forgive is the very wound we are bringing to Jesus, we can be absolutely sure of his help, because to forgive is the thing that most pleases him, and he will never refuse his compassion when our hurt seems too great for us to forgive. He knows our hurt from experience, yet he forgave, freely and utterly.

> *"It is a credit to you if, aware of God, you endure*
> *pain while suffering unjustly . . . If you endure*
> *when you do right and suffer for it, you have God's*
> *approval. For to this you have been called, because*
> *Christ also suffered for you, leaving you an*
> *example, so that you should follow in his steps. He*
> *committed no sin, and no lie was found in his*
> *mouth. When he was abused, he did not retaliate;*
> *when he suffered, he did not threaten; but he*
> *entrusted himself to the one who judges justly."*
>
> 1 PT 2:19-23

Inner healing of the emotions depends to a great extent on reconciliation with God. It depends on repentance for sins and God's consequent forgiveness of those sins. Repentance and acceptance of God's mercy in reconciliation with him is a kind of inner healing, a spiritual healing. And it is closely connected with emotional healing and can often lead to it. On the other hand, little healing of the emotions by the power of the Holy Spirit is possible unless repentance and reconciliation with God are present.

However, the grace of repentance frequently depends on my forgiving others. God can forgive us only insofar as we forgive others; and so we pray "forgive us our trespasses as we forgive those who trespass against us." If I do not forgive others, the hurt or bitterness, or resentment, or anger inside me keeps me from that repentance and openness to God that are necessary for my acceptance of God's forgiveness and so for the healing of my emotions and feelings.

Sometimes our failure to forgive is buried, lies below

the level of awareness. We think, or we take for granted, that we have forgiven others; but our resentment and unforgiveness remain inside us, not conscious. This is why it is often important to forgive those who have hurt us, whether they intended to or not, even when we are not aware of any bitterness or lack of forgiveness on our part.

And many of us need to forgive ourselves for our sins, our mistakes and our failures. I need to accept Jesus' and the Father's total and unconditional acceptance of me; accepting God's acceptance of me, I can accept myself. Our Lord loves me not in spite of the dark side of myself but partly because of it; he came to save not the just but sinners, and my sinfulness attracts his loving compassion. Accepting his compassionate and loving forgiveness and acceptance of me, I can forgive myself.

Sometimes we need to forgive God. Obviously, there is no fault at all in God. Nevertheless, I might feel, in a vague way, some resentment against God for my own limitations or failures, for illness or an accident, for the death of someone I love, or for circumstances of my life. God wants me to forgive him, so that I can get over my resentment, accept his love better, and be healed.

Praying for Inner Healing

Perhaps now, reading this chapter, or later in a moment of tranquillity, you can pray for inner healing.

1. The first step is to ask, with as much faith as you have, that the Lord heal you interiorly:

Lord, you have told us to ask and we will receive, to seek and we will find, to knock and you will open the door to us. I ask you now for inner

healing. Heal me, make me whole. I trust in your
personal love for me and in the healing power of
your compassion.

2. The second step is repentance, a turning to the Lord for forgiveness. Coming into the light of his love and understanding, I am free to see myself as I really am and to become more aware of the sin, the disorder, and the hurts and the wounds inside me. I am free, in the Lord's love, to see better my need for forgiveness and for inner healing.

Lord, I am sorry for all my sins, and I trust in your
mercy. With your help, I renounce my sins and any
sinful patterns in my life; I renounce everything
that in any way opposes you. I accept with all my
heart your forgiving love. And I ask you for the
grace to be aware of the disorder in my inner self,
to experience my own interior disorder with my
wounds and hurts and sinfulness.

Guide me in this prayer; show me what to pray for
and how to pray. Bring to my mind whatever pain
or hurts you want me to ask you to heal.

3. Now, see what problem or painful experience comes to mind, and pray for healing regarding that problem or that memory. (If more that one thing comes to mind, take them one at a time.) It might be a failure or a broken friendship or the loss of a person you love. It could be something in childhood, such as a less than perfect relationship with your father or your mother. It could be present anger or depression or some undesirable behavior pattern.

Pray in your own words, lifting up the hurt or the

painful memory or the problem to the Lord for healing. Pray simply like a child.

4. Forgive everyone involved, praying for them by name and telling the Lord that, with his help, you forgive each one. Imagine the person to be forgiven and, in your imagination, put your arms around that person and say, "I forgive you." Then see the Lord in your imagination, his arms outstretched to embrace you both, and — with one arm around the person you have forgiven — walk with that person into the Lord's arms and let him forgive you both and reconcile you to each other and to himself.

5. Picture in your imagination the situation the problem goes back to. Or the place of the hurtful memory. Picture the Lord in that place and situation, filling it with his healing love, being with you there. And ask him to heal you, again praying simply and in your own words.

Inner Healing in Context

Inner healing can take place in personal prayer when a person prays alone; it can take place while praying for inner healing with one or two other persons; and it can take place in a group where inner healing is prayed for. Privileged situations for healing to take place are the sacraments, especially Reconciliation, the Anointing of the Sick and the Eucharist, celebration of the Lord's supper. When I confess my sins, I can express sorrow for them, receive God's pardon and his peace, and also pray for and receive healing of the wounds and hurts that might be connected with the sins I confessed or that might be at the root of the sinful tendencies that resulted in those sins. The sacrament of the Anointing of the Sick is not only in preparation for the life to come, but for forgiveness of sins and for both bodily and inner healing. The Eucharist, especially, is the sacrament of the healing of personal relationships, of being made more one in Jesus through sharing the same bread. And, in general, the prayer, ". . . but only say the word and I shall be healed" is meant to be said in faith, with a faith that is hopeful, that *expects* (for hope is expectation in faith) healing to take place.

So far we have considered inner healing somewhat as an isolated action, a result of an explicit prayer for healing. Inner healing can also be situated within the total process of encountering the Lord; seen in this way, inner healing can be understood more realistically. Furthermore, it can be understood better as an integral part of growth in union with the Lord, as a condition of deep conversion, and as leading to service.

The story of the meeting between Jesus and the Samaritan woman (Jn 4:7-42) casts light on the place of inner healing as part of the process of prayer. The process begins with a journey, a movement towards the Lord, ending with a stopping short in his presence. There takes place a bringing to awareness of the disorder in the woman's life and the beginning of a re-ordering. This incipient re-ordering itself initiates a conversion process that clarified the woman's understanding of herself — as a sinner and as called. In turn, conversion brings her closer to the Lord and gives her a new freedom which takes shape in mission; she goes out to the other Samaritans with the good news, having accepted a call that names her personally and that goes beyond that, to become a call to go to others, a sending to bring the good news of the Lord. The Samaritan woman understands better who she is *("He told me all I ever did.")* in her acceptance of Jesus *("Could he be the Christ?"),* and she goes out to spread the good news *("Come and see . . .").*

The healing of Peter's mother-in-law (Mk 1:29-31) shows the same connection between healing and service *(The fever left her; and she served them)*. The received healing becomes a new freedom to serve. It occurs commonly, when a person receives a healing from the Lord, that the person looks for some form of service to give shape to his gratitude and to his freedom.

᳐

Two

The Truth of Myself and the Mercy of the Lord

Mary's Magnificat

MARY, greeting her pregnant cousin Elizabeth, and carrying Jesus in her womb, says:

> "My soul magnifies the Lord,
> my spirit is glad in God my Savior;
> because he has looked with favor
> on the lowliness of his servant."

LK 1:46-48

Mary magnifies God. She glorifies him, praises him, gives him glory. Mary acts as a focus for the Lord, in analogy with a magnifying glass that focuses the sun's rays. Praise results, praise that glorifies, magnifies God. Why? Because she is humble before the Lord. Considering herself a servant, a handmaid, Mary lowers herself, humbles herself. She stands, humble, before the Lord in the truth of her own existence: that she depends entirely on God and on his merciful love for her. She depends on the Lord for her very existence, for her role as the mother of Jesus, for everything. The recognition in Mary's heart of this reality, of this factual state of affairs, is her humility, her lowliness.

Clear from the gospels, and manifest in the entire Christian tradition of writing and painting, is this: that Mary's outstanding quality, her great virtue, is her humility before God, her openness, her transparency before the Lord. The highest of human beings — because she is the mother of God — comes to Elizabeth, and to everyone, including God, as the lowest, the most humble. The first becomes the lowest, the last. And that is why she is the first, why she finds favor with God. The Lord looks on Mary with favor because she is lowly.

Mary's humility before God comes from her knowledge of her creatureliness. Even though sinless from her conception, even though the Mother of God, Mary remains completely a creature. We surely do not have Mary's great humility, but we do have more reason for it in our sins and our sinfulness.

Another figure in Luke's gospel who finds favor with God is the publican, the tax collector, in Jesus' parable.

The Pharisee and the Tax Collector

Jesus tells the story, the parable, of two men who go to the temple to pray, a pharisee and a tax collector, a publican.

> *"Two men went up to the temple to pray, a pharisee and a publican. The pharisee stood and prayed like this, 'God, I thank thee that I am not as other men are, cheaters, unjust, adulterers, or even like this*

> *publican. I fast twice a week, I give money to the*
> *temple.' The publican, standing afar off, would not*
> *lift up so much as his eyes to heaven, but struck his*
> *breast saying, 'God, be merciful to me a sinner.' I*
> *tell you this man went down to his house justified*
> *rather than the other, for everyone that exalts*
> *himself shall be abased, and he that humbles himself*
> *shall be raised up."*
>
> LK 18:10-14

The pharisee is not a bad man. He is a good man, a model of traditional human holiness. He fasts more than the law requires. He prays for others. He gives money to the synagogue. He thanks God for God's mercy on him. When the pharisee prays, he surely follows the standard way of praying at that time in the Jewish religion: he lifts his arms and his eyes to heaven, and he prays out loud.

The publican on the other hand, the tax collector, is a thoroughly bad man. He works for the Roman troops that occupy the city of Jerusalem. He collects taxes for them; that is, he takes money from his fellow Jews and gives it to the occupying army. Since Israel was a theocracy, uniting civil government and religion, the tax collector betrays his fellow countrymen, his country, and his religion and his God. He could not be worse.

And he refuses to pray correctly. He does not lift eyes or hands to heaven. He does not call on God's name. In anguish of heart, he calls out to God, "Lord, have mercy on me a sinner." He is desperate and lost.

But does not the publican become converted in the temple? No. He cannot change his life without losing his job, his livelihood. He remains an unconverted sinner, a lost soul.

But the publican, not the pharisee, finds favor with God. The publican, not the pharisee, goes home justified before God. Why? Why the tax collector, a bad man? And why not the good man, the pharisee?

The publican knows who he is, a sinner. He recognizes his nothingness before God, his total dependence on God and on God's mercy. He finds favor with God partly because he is a sinner and recognizes his sinfulness. The fact of his weakness and sinfulness attracts the Lord's compassion; God's compassion is an integral part of his love. The Lord loves the publican not in spite of his weakness and sinfulness, but partly because of it, and because the publican knows his own sinfulness and weakness and misery. He knows who he is before God: a sinner.

Jesus actually seems to prefer the company of sinners. When he eats at the table of a pharisee, at the home of Simon the pharisee for example, Jesus does not seem entirely at ease. He chooses the home of the publican Zaccheus as a place to spend the night.

When the pharisees complain to Jesus about his having table fellowship with publicans and prostitutes, he tells them that it is not the healthy that need the doctor, but those who are ill. He tells the pharisees to learn the meaning of the prophetic saying "I want mercy, not sacrifice" (Hos 6:6; Mt 9:10-13). And that he, Jesus, has come not to call the virtuous but sinners.

The pharisees are really ill and spiritually blind, but they complacently consider themselves healthy. They put themselves beyond help from the "doctor" because they do not admit their illness.

Spiritual Blindness

In the Old Testament, in the book of the prophet Isaiah, Israel's leaders have spiritual blindness because they are selfish, greedy, and lazy (Is 56:10). This makes them blind to God's truth:

> *"Be stupid and stunned, be blind. . . . God has*
> *made the prophets blind, he has covered the eyes of*
> *the seers."*
>
> IS 29:9-10

They are blind to even their own spiritual blindness:

> *"Make the eyes of this people blind so that they*
> *cannot see; if they did see, they might turn to me*
> *and be healed."*
>
> IS 6:10

Spiritual blindness is the culpable inability to see the true and the good that God reveals in our lives. Usually, spiritual blindness is attributed to righteous and respectable people. This blindness comes about either as a sin, or as a result of sin.

In the New Testament, self righteousness and hypocrisy result in spiritual blindness. Paul admonishes those who call themselves Jews:

> *"You have confidence that you are guides for the*
> *blind, a light for those in darkness, instructors for*
> *the foolish and teachers for the ignorant; why don't*
> *you teach yourselves?"*
>
> ROM 2:19-23

They preach, *"Do not steal,"* but they steal; they teach to not commit adultery, but they do it themselves.

Worldliness can cause spiritual blindness:

> *"The evil god of this world keeps them from seeing*
> *the light that shines on them."*
>
> 2 COR 4:4

So can the absence of Christian virtues: knowledge, faith, goodness, self-control, endurance, godliness, brotherly love . . . . *Whoever does not have these is blind, he cannot see* (2 Pt 1:9).

Again, spiritual blindness makes us blind to our own blindness. The Apocalypse tells the church in Laodicea that it says to itself *"I am rich and well off, and I have everything I need,"* but it does not recognize its own misery. *"You are poor and blind and naked"* (Rev 3:17).

Jesus speaks to the scribes and the pharisees:

> *"Blind guides! You hypocrites, . . . blind fools, . . . how blind you are. You neglect justice and mercy and honesty; these you should practice without neglecting the others. Blind guides, . . . clean the inside of the cup and then the outside will be clean too. You are like tombs; you appear good on the outside, but inside you are full of hypocrisy and sins."*
>
> MT 23:23-28

> *"Blind leaders of the blind, . . . both fall into the ditch."*
>
> MT 15:14

> *"You hypocrites, take the log out of your own eye, then you will be able to see the speck in your brother's eye."*
>
> LK 6:41

The Johannine writings consider spiritual blindness within the framework of light and darkness. Love and light go together, opposed to lack of love and to darkness (cf. 1Jn 2:11). Jesus uses the words of Deutero-Isaiah (Is 6:10):

> *"God has blinded their eyes and closed their minds so that they would not turn to me for healing."*
>
> JN 12:20

In the First Letter to the Corinthians, Saint Paul criticizes the Corinthian Christians severely, putting emphasis on their pride, on their being puffed up. The Romans had destroyed the Greek city of Corinth in the year 146 BC. The Roman Emperor Julius Caesar rebuilt the city, and it became an important port, cosmopolitan, with people of many nationalities.

Paul wrote this letter because he had heard about the Corinthians' problems from a certain Chloe: misunderstandings arising from a previous (now lost) letter, the immorality of the Corinthian Christians, their divisions, their legal problems with one another, the confusion in their Eucharistic celebrations and other prayer assemblies, their lack of love for one another, and because they thought they were "spiritual."

In Chapters Four, Five, and Six, Paul writes about pride, about being puffed up with pride, and its consequences. The Corinthian Christians are *puffed up* (4:6, 4:18-19, 5:2; 8:1; 13:4). They think that they are spiritual *(pneumatikoi* in the Greek), but they are really puffed up with hot air *(phousiousthe)*. In fact, the Greek word *phousiousthe* means flatulent. Somewhat vulgarly, Paul makes a play on words; in Greek, the two words for "spiritual" and "puffed up" are similar. Paul tells the Corinthians that they think themselves spiritual. However, the spirit in them is not the Holy Spirit but hot air. They are not spiritual, they are flatulent.

The word flatulence in this letter to Corinth has a metaphorical role. It means: puffed up with the hot air of pride, of self importance, of complacency, of arrogance. This is, of course, the pride that results in spiritual blindness. Paul wants to shock the Corinthian Christians out of their complacent consideration of themselves as wonderful and spirit-filled Christians. They are not, he tells them, filled with the Spirit at all; what they are filled with is quite something else. Pride.

And so no wonder that the Corinthian Christians are blind to their own misery. They have serious spiritual blindness. So not just the Jews, but Christians too can get complacent, puffed up, full of the hot air of blinding pride.

In the New Testament, and especially in the Johannine writings, physical blindness often has a metaphorical or somehow symbolic aspect. After the healing of the man born blind, and after the Pharisees have refused to accept the fact of the man's healing, Jesus says: *"I have come into the world so that the blind might see and that those who see might become blind"* (Jn 9:39). The Pharisees ask him if they are blind. He replies, *"If you were blind, you would not be guilty, but because you say, 'We see,' your guilt remains"* (Jn 9:39-41).

The Bible describes messianic salvation as the healing of blindness, as light to the blind; Jesus quotes the Book of Isaiah (61:1-2), *"He has sent me . . . to bring sight to the blind"* (Lk 4:18). The Book of Revelation advises the blind church of Laodicea to *"buy from me . . . ointment to put on your eyes so that you may see"* (3:18). And it specifies the precise remedy for spiritual blindness: conversion of heart, *"Repent in earnest; behold, I stand at the door and knock"* (3:19-20). The Lord wants me to receive his mercy. The door's handle is on my side. Only I can open the door.

Spiritual blindness, then, finds healing through the grace of conversion, and this comes about through the mercy of God. Thomas Aquinas states that only by divine mercy can spiritual blindness be healed.[1] Spiritual blindness comes about through holding on to evil and resisting the light of God. God withholds the light of his grace from those in whom he finds serious obstacles, and it is in this sense only that we can speak of God causing spiritual blindness.[2] The acceptance of the Lord's mercy depends on my accepting myself as a sinner.

I Can Glory in My Infirmities

In the parable of the prodigal son who takes his inheritance and leaves home, spending all his money and ending in destitution and misery, and finally returning home repentant to accept his father's mercy, Jesus tells us about his attitude — and his Father's attitude — toward sinners who recognize their own sinfulness and misery. And Jesus adds to the main story: the story of the older of the two brothers, who becomes angry when the Father welcomes the younger son back home with a celebration and with lavish mercy. The difference between the two sons is that the younger has hit bottom; he knows who he is, a poor sinner. The elder son thinks himself good and worthy; he does not know that he too is a poor sinner.

When I discover my poverty before the Lord, I find his favor. When I recognize that I am a poor sinner, miserable in my sinfulness, and turn to him, I find him there waiting for me with mercy. I find access to the Lord's heart.

The Lord loves me not in spite of the fact that I am weak and a sinner, but partly because of that very fact. My weakness and my sinfulness, acknowledged by me, form the opening in me to the Lord's love. His love is compassionate, merciful, by its nature. Compassion stands as one of the integral components of the Lord's love for me. His love for me entails no finger wagging on his part; he does not demand that I become better before he will love me more. He loves me to the maximum now. With no conditions, and with no qualifications.

So, with Saint Paul, I can glory in my infirmities, in my sinfulness and my weakness, because God's merciful and compassionate love is made perfect in my weakness. This is the beginning of inner healing.

Lord Jesus, you know me perfectly. You know my good qualities and my bad ones. You know my past; you see it clearly. You know my future; you see it happening. You love me just as I am, without any conditions, without any qualifications.

You do not condemn me. You do not judge me. You do forgive me. You have given your life for me on the cross as though I were the only other person besides you who ever walked on earth, and you would do it again if you had to. You call me by name, and you love me.

Jesus, free me from my pride, my complacency, my search for the glory of this world and for attention and prestige and appreciation. Teach me humility.

Heal me of any spiritual blindness, Lord, that I may see your face with the eyes of faith, with the eyes of my heart. Teach me to know you through love, especially for the powerful and personal love that you have in your heart for me.

Thank you for your love for me. Amen.

THREE

Crying Out to the Lord

FROM THE CROSS, Jesus cries out to the Father, "Eloi, Eloi, lama sabachthani?" (*"My God, my God, why have you forsaken me?"* Mk 15:34; Mt 27:46); he prays from the heart, expressing how he feels. Completely broken down, dying, incapable or putting words together to form a prayer, he falls back on a prayer he knows by heart, and speaks the first verse of Psalm 22. Psalm 22 well expresses Jesus' situation on the cross. It is a prayer that fits so well as to be prophetic of the passion.

> *"But I am a worm, and not human;*
> *scorned by others, and despised by the people.*
> *All who see me mock me;*
> *they make mouths at me, they shake their heads:*
> *'Commit your cause to the Lord;*
> *let him deliver — let him rescue the one*
> *in whom he delights'."* (vv.6-8)
> *"They have pierced my hands and my feet."* (v.16)
> *"They divide my clothes among themselves,*
> *and for my clothing they cast lots."* (v.18)

The gospel writers, aware of Jesus' suffering and death as fulfilling the scriptures, consciously point out the fulfillment of Psalm 22. But this hardly accounts for the prayer of Jesus' agony; he prays, not to prove that he fulfills prophecies, but to cry out to God. He laments, complains, cries out to his Father for deliverance — not with despair, but in extreme distress. The answer to Jesus' cry, his deliverance, comes in the resurrection.

Psalm 22 is a prayer of lament, a kind of prayer that, sadly, we neglect in Christianity.[1]

Psalms of Lament

Several psalms are lamentations, prayers of lament. They reflect the way we instinctively pray when we are suffering. Usually they begin with a cry to God: *"My God, my God"* (Ps 22:1); *"Save me O God"* (Ps 69:1); *"Have mercy on me O God"* (Ps 51:1); *"O God, why have you cast us off?"* (Ps 74:1); *"Out of the depths I am calling to you Lord"* (Ps 130:1); *"As a deer thirsts for running streams, so my soul longs for you, O God"* (Ps 42:1). Psalm 102 has a longer introduction:

> *"Hear my prayer, O Lord, let my cry come to you!*
> *Do not hide your face from me*
> *in the day of my distress!*
> *Turn your ear to me;*
> *answer me speedily in the day when I call."* (vv.1-2)

There follows a description of the situation — telling God in detail what the trouble is, and lamenting, complaining to God. For example, Psalm 22 continues:

> *"Why have you forsaken me?*
> *O my God, I cry by day, but you do not answer;*
> *and by night, but find no rest."* (vv.1-2)

And it goes on to detail the plight of the suffering one:

"I am poured out like water . . .
my strength is dried up like a potsherd . . .
you lay me in the dust of death." (vv.14-15)

"I pour out my complaint before him;
I tell my trouble before him."

PS.142:2

"My heart is in anguish within me,
the terrors of death have fallen upon me."

PS 55:4

"Those who would destroy me attack me with lies.
What I did not steal must I now pay back?"

PS 69:4

"You have made the earth quake,
you have torn it open."

PS 60:2

"Your hand has come down on me.
There is no health in my flesh."

PS 38: 2-3

Psalm 69 begins:

"Save me, O God,
for the waters have come up to my neck.
I sink in deep mire, where there is no foothold;
I have come into deep waters,
and the flood sweeps over me.
I am weary with crying; my throat is parched.
My eyes grow dim with waiting
for my God." (vv.1-3)

In Jerusalem is the house of Caiaphas, the high priest at the time of Jesus' death. Here is a pit into which the condemned man was thrown until his execution. We know that Jesus spent his last night at the house of Caiaphas (Jn 18:28). Jesus might well have made his own the lament of Psalm 88:

> *"O Lord, God of my salvation,*
> *when at night I cry out in your presence,*
> *let my prayer come before you; incline your ear to*
> *my cry.*
> *For my soul is full of troubles, and my life draws*
> *near to Sheol.*
> *I am counted among those who go down to the Pit;*
> *I am like those who have no help . . . like those you*
> *have forgotten . . .*
> *You have put me in the depth of the Pit. . . .*
> *You have caused my companions to shun me;*
> *I am shut in so that I cannot escape . . .*
> *you have made me a thing of horror to them."*

And Psalm 44, after describing in some detail the trouble the psalmist finds himself in, and after complaining strongly to God, finally shouts: *"Wake up! Why O Lord are you asleep? Wake up!"* (v.23)

Having cried out and lamented, the psalm-prayer always trusts. Almost always this trust appears as an act of will, unfelt in the emotions. The psalmist says he will cling to God even if he feels no better.

> *"Why are you cast down my soul?*
> *Why are you troubled within me?*
> *Hope in God . . . my helper and my God."*

PS 42:5-6

> *"You are holy, enthroned on the praises of Israel.*
> *In you our ancestors trusted;*

they trusted and you delivered them.
To you they cried, and were saved;
they trusted in you and were not put to shame."

PS 22:3-5

"I wait for the Lord, my soul waits,
and in his word I hope;
My soul waits for the Lord more than watchmen
for the morning,
more than watchmen for the dawn."

PS 130:3-7

Confidence crystallizes in petition. The extreme distress is still there, but not despair. Trust is calmer, though pressing, as the psalmist urges:

"Come quickly to my aid."

PS 22:19

"Do not let the pit close its mouth over me."

PS 69:15

"Send out your light and your truth,
let them lead me."

PS 43:3

"Bring me out of prison."

PS 142:7

"In your steadfast righteousness,
bring me out of trouble."

PS 143:11

"O God, deal on my behalf for thy name's sake . . .
For I am poor . . . my heart is stricken."

PS 109:21-22

The psalm of lament cries out, complains, trusts, asks.

Usually the conclusion is a promise to give witness to the way the Lord rescues and saves.

> *"My tongue will sing aloud of your deliverance."*
>
> PS 51:14

> *"I will magnify him with thanksgiving."*
>
> PS 69:30

> *"My lips will shout for joy*
> *when I sing praises to thee:*
> *my soul also which thou hast rescued.*
> *And my tongue will talk of thy righteous help*
> *all the day long."*
>
> PS 71:23-24

> *"With my mouth I will give great thanks*
> *to the Lord.*
> *I will praise him in the midst of the throng;*
> *for he stands at the right hand of the needy."*
>
> PS 109:30-31

The psalm of lament, then, does not stop at lamentation. It complains to God, but then transcends any tendency to self-pity by appealing to him who can remove the suffering. The complaint moves into a trustful turning to the Lord and so into asking to be saved. The psalm of lament is a prayer for healing that ends in thanking and praising God for his healing power. This final praise and thanksgiving indicate that an interior change takes place in the course of the prayer, that the beginning of healing takes place or is at least implied right in the prayer itself.

Lament in the Old Testament

The psalms of lament form the heart of the Old Testament tradition of lament, and contain most of its highly developed expressions. However, the prayer of lament is an integral part of the prayer tradition of the whole Old Testament. The two basic categories of Old Testament piety, covenant and exodus, give the people of Israel the right to lament — because God is their God and they are his people — and establish lament to God as the beginning of salvation. The Exodus begins with the Lord's response to the crying out of his people.

Perhaps the oldest text in the Bible, the certainly ancient cultic formula of Deuteronomy 26:5-10, contains a summary of the Exodus experience in the form of a prayer of gratitude:

> *"A wandering Aramean was my father; and he went down into Egypt and lived there, few in number; and he became a nation, great, powerful, and populous. And the Egyptians treated us harshly, and afflicted us, and laid upon us hard bondage. Then we cried to the Lord, the God of our fathers, and the Lord heard us, and saw our affliction, our toil, and our oppression; and the Lord brought us out of Egypt with a mighty hand and an outstretched arm, with great terror, with signs and wonders; and he brought us into this place and gave us this land, a land flowing with milk and honey. And behold, now I bring the first of the fruit of the ground, which you, O Lord, have given me."*

This summary of the first fifteen chapters of the Book of Exodus situates the place of the prayer of lament in the spirituality of the Old Testament and underlines its significance. *"Then we cried to the Lord,"* this phrase establishes the Exodus itself as a response to prayer, to the cry of the people of God for help. The anguished cry for help, more than an historical event, constitutes a dimension of Israel's relationship with God; lament is an important part of what happens between God and his people in the history of the covenant relationship. Over and over in Israel's history, the people cry out to the Lord, and he hears their voice and sees their affliction and *is moved to compassion by their groaning* (Jgs 2:18).

The pattern is always the same: people, in suffering and anguish, cry out to the Lord for help; the Lord hears their cry and brings them out of their suffering and into a new and blessed situation; the people rejoice in the Lord, praising and thanking him. Cain laments: *"My punishment is greater than I can bear"* and the Lord answers, *"Not so,"* and puts a saving mark on him (Gen 4:13). Hagar and her son lament; the Lord hears the boy weeping and reassures Hagar: *and God was with the lad, and he grew up* (Gen 21:16-20). Samson, ready to die of thirst, calls on the Lord; water gushes out of a hollow place, *and when he drank, his spirit returned, and he revived* (Jgs 15:18-19). When the tribe of Benjamin seems lost to Israel, the people lift up their voices to God, and weep bitterly before him (Jgs 21:2), and he answers their prayer. Hannah cries out to God, weeping bitterly, complaining of her inability to have a child; *and the Lord remembered her; and in due time Hannah conceived and bore a son, and she named him Samuel* (1 Sam 1:10-20). Samuel explaining to the people that the Lord has given them Saul as king, recounts the times Israel cried out and was delivered by the Lord: *". . . your fathers cried to the Lord, and the Lord sent Moses and Aaron, who led your fathers out of Egypt . . . And they cried to the Lord, and the Lord sent Jerubaal and Barak, and Jephthah, and Samson, and delivered you"* (1 Sam 12:8-11). Solomon, praying at the dedication of the temple, asks the Lord to hear any laments of the people offered in the temple, and to forgive their sins, save them from their afflictions, and restore them to well-being (2 Chr 6:24-31).

The outstanding example of individual lamentation is the Book of Job. Job's lament consists of bitter complaining to God against God. He refuses his friends' ideas that his suffering is a punishment for sin or that it has any rational explanation. He has no way to understand his situation; it is absurd, and the philosophical arguments of Job's friends only highlight the absurdity. Finally, the Lord responds to Job, and Job declares humbly to God that he has spoken about matters to deep for him, and that he repents *in dust and ashes* (Jb 42:1-6). *And the Lord restored the fortunes of Job* (Jb 42:10).

The lament for the people, for the nation, is a common form of prayer of lament. Psalms 79 and 80 are psalms of lament for Israel, begging the Lord for his own name's sake for forgiveness and liberation (79:9), not to be angry for ever (79:5; 80:4), but to let his face shine that his people may be saved (80:3,7 and 19). The exodus begins with a lament of the people that the Lord listens to:

> *"Then the Lord said, 'I have seen the suffering of*
> *my people who are in Egypt, and have heard their*
> *cry because of their taskmasters . . .'"*
>
> EX 3:7

And lament continues during the exodus in the form of the murmuring of the people. National prayers of lament are frequent throughout Israel's history; they ask for deliverance from enemy forces, from natural disasters, and for the restoration of Israel. For example, the people of Judah lament to the Lord:

> *"Look down from heaven and see . . .*
> *Where are your zeal and your power?*
> *The yearning of your heart and your compassion*
> *are held from me."*
>
> IS 63:15; the whole prayer is IS 63:15-64:12

A special type of national lament is the prayer of lament for the people by a mediator. The mediator cries out to God for his or her people, and becomes instrumental in God's saving response to that prayer of lament. Moses laments, complains to God, prays for God's people in Exodus:

> "O Lord, why does your wrath burn hot
> against your people . . .?
> Why should the Egyptians say, 'With evil intent
> he brought them forth,
> to slay them in the mountains' . . .?"

The text continues: *And the Lord repented of the evil which he thought to do to his people.* (Ex 32:11-14. See also Dt 9:25-29; Ex 32:30-32; Ex 33:12-19; Nm 11:1-23; 12:13; 14:11-19; Jos 7:6-9). Gideon complains to the angel of the Lord, who has told him that the Lord is with him:

> " 'But sir, if the Lord is with us, why has all this
> happened to us? And where are all his wonderful
> deeds which our ancestors recounted to us?' . . .
> And the Lord turned to him and said, 'Go in this
> might of yours and deliver Israel from the hand of
> Midian; do I not send you?' And he responded,
> 'But Lord, how can I deliver Israel? My clan is the
> weakest in Manasseh, and I am the least in my
> family.' And the Lord said to him, 'But I will be
> with you . . .' "

JGS 6:13-16

David, conscious that his people are suffering the plague because of David's own sin, speaks to the Lord:

> "I alone have sinned and I alone have done
> wickedly; but these sheep, what have they done?"

1 CHR 21:17

He offers burnt offerings and peace offerings, and the plague is averted. At the moment of the evening incense offering in the Jerusalem temple, Judith, prostrate, cries out in a loud voice to the Lord in a beautiful prayer of lament for her people:

> *". . . for you have done these things and those that
> went before, and those that followed after. You have
> designed the things that are now . . . what you had
> in mind has happened; the things you decided on
> presented themselves and said 'Here we are.' . . .
> but you are the God of the lowly, helper of the
> oppressed, upholder of the weak . . . you are the
> God of all power . . . there is no other who protects
> the people of Israel but you alone!"*
>
> JDT 9:5-6;11-12

The Lord uses Judith to deliver Israel in a victory that she celebrates in a joyful canticle of praise and thanksgiving (Jdt 15:14-16:17). Daniel seeks the Lord *by prayer and supplications with fasting and sackcloth and ashes, praying for forgiveness and salvation for the people* (Dn 9:3-19). Ezra pleads for the people, newly re-established in Israel after their exile (Ez 9:1-2; Neh 9:6-37). One of the most beautiful prayers of lament on behalf of the community is the last chapter of Jeremiah's Lamentations; it ends in a prayer for reconciliation and inner healing:

> *"Alas that we ever sinned!
> At this our heart has become sick;
> These things have darkened our sight.
> On Mount Zion, lying desolate, foxes prowl.
> Yet you Lord, rule for ever;
> Your throne is eternal.
> Why do you never think of us?
> Why abandon us so long?
> Bring us back to you, Lord, and we will return.*

Make our days as they were before.
But instead you have completely rejected us;
You have been very angry with us."

LAM 5:16-22[2]

The mediator prays, cries out, that the people be saved, and then, somehow, becomes part of the process of salvation. This is clearest in the case of the Suffering Servant of Deutero Isaiah, (chapters 44ff.) who answers Israel's complaint that, *"The Lord has forsaken me, my Lord has forgotten me"* (Is 49:14) with a message of consoling hope and with a suffering intercession that *"bears the sin of many, and makes intercession for the transgressors"* (Is 53:12).

The passion and death of Jesus follow in detail the songs of the Suffering Servant, with whom Jesus explicitly identifies himself, particularly in his predictions of his suffering and death. The long Old Testament tradition of the mediator's prayer of lament for the people, a tradition culminating in the laments of Jeremiah and in the mediation of the Suffering Servant of Second Isaiah, is gathered up in the intercessory act of Jesus in laying down his life.

The Nature of the Prayer of Lament

Three things need to be observed about the tradition of lament in the Old Testament. The first is that the lament is hopeful; it looks to the future, to liberation, to healing. It is not a lament of mourning or regret that looks backwards to past loss or failure, but a lament of affliction that cries out to God for freedom from the affliction.

Secondly, the prayer of lament knows no reasons. No attempt is made to argue for deliverance on the basis of the merits of the afflicted. The appeal is directly to the Lord's compassion. The need is shown him; he is simply asked to look at the wounds, at the suffering, and to act in his loving mercy and faithful compassion. The Lord acts because of his own goodness, his own holiness.

> *"Thus says the Lord God: 'It is not for your sake,*
> *O house of Israel, that I am about to act, but for the*
> *sake of my holy name. . . . I will sprinkle clean*
> *water upon you, and you shall be clean from all*
> *your uncleannesses; and from all our idols I will*
> *cleanse you. A new heart I will give you, and a new*
> *spirit I will put within you; and I will take out of*
> *your flesh the heart of stone and give you a heart of*
> *flesh. And I will put my spirit within you. . . .' "*
>
> EZK 36:22-27

And his action in response to cries for help is to save and to heal — both physically and interiorly — not only to forgive sins.

Finally, something must be said about the place of sin in the prayer of lament. The salvation asked for is rarely salvation from sin. Sometimes, however, it is, as in Psalm 51, *"Have mercy on me O God,"* the great prayer for forgiveness and spiritual healing, and in David's prayer for forgiveness of his sin (2 Sam 24:10). The prayer of lament asks for salvation *now,* for help in this life, for freedom from enemies, for the healing of sickness, for deliverance from hunger and thirst. This fact has important implications for our understanding of prayer for inner healing and for our understanding of the meaning of the salvation that Jesus Christ won for us through his suffering and death.

Prayer of Lament in the New Testament

The most common prayer of lament in the gospels is the request, made to Jesus, for healing.

"And a leper came to him, and kneeling said to
him, 'If you will, you can make me clean.' Moved
with compassion, he stretched out his hand and
touched him, and said to him, 'I will; be clean.'
And immediately the leprosy left him, and he was
made clean."

MK 1:40-42

The Canaanite woman begs Jesus for the healing of her daughter (Mk 7:25-30), Bartimaeus, the blind beggar, cries out: *"Jesus, Son of David, have mercy on me"* over and over (Mk 10:46-52), just as the ten lepers call out: *"Jesus, Master, have mercy on us"* (Lk 17:12-19). After Lazarus' death, Martha tells Jesus: *"Lord, if you had been here, my brother would not have died. And even now I know that whatever you ask from God, God will give you"* (Jn 11:21-22).

Often, the "prayer of lament" is simply the silent presence of suffering, either physical, as in the cure of Peter's mother-in-law's fever (Mk 1:30-31), or spiritual as well as physical, as in the forgiveness and healing of the paralytic lowered by his friends through a hole in the roof (Mk 2:3-12). Jesus sees the widow of Nain, has compassion on her, tells her not to weep, and raises up her dead son (Lk 7:12-15).

Jesus, in his teaching on prayer, encourages asking with faith and expecting to receive a positive answer to prayer of petition (e.g., Mt 6:7-12; Jn 16:23-24). The parable of the unrighteous judge has as its point the efficacy of crying out to God; Jesus makes it explicit:

"And will not God vindicate his elect, who cry to
him day and night? Will he delay long over them?
I tell you, he will vindicate them speedily."

LK 18:1-8

Jesus himself cries out in lament to the Father in his

agony in the garden and in praying the first verse of Psalm 22 on the cross. His other laments, however, seem to be in line with the Old Testament tradition of the lament of God. God laments for his people especially in the prophecies of Jeremiah (see 8:5-7; 12:7-13; 15:5-9; 18:13-17). At the beginning of the book of Isaiah, God complains: *"Sons I have reared and brought up, but they have rebelled against me"* (1:2). The whole book of Hosea is based on God's lament over his people:

> *"The Lord said to Hosea, 'Go, take a prostitute for a wife, because the country is committing fornication by forsaking the Lord'."*
>
> HOSEA 1:2

This tradition of God lamenting over his people, his disappointment and anger expressed to Moses during the Exodus (e.g., Num 14:11), down through the prophetic books, seems to find its final expression in the laments of God become man. Jesus weeps over Jerusalem:

> *"How often would I have gathered your children together as a hen gathers her brood under her wings, and you would not! Behold, your house is forsaken."*
>
> LK 13:34-35

He laments its future destruction (Lk 21:23). He complains about the lack of faith of his disciples (e.g., Mt 17:17), and he upbraids cities that will not repent.

Crying Out to the Lord

When we need help, we can, and should, cry out to the Lord, not afraid to express how we feel, openly speaking to him our pain or resentment or fear or sadness. One way to come to the Lord lamenting is to choose a prayer of lament from the Psalms, or from some other book in the Old Testament, and say it slowly with the present situation in mind. Another way is to pray in your own words, following the structure of the psalms of lament:

1. Calling out to the Lord; for example, *"Jesus, Son of David, have mercy on me"* or *"Out of the depths I cry to you O Lord."*

2. Lamenting, complaining, expressing just how you feel to the Lord.

3. An act of trust, of confidence in the Lord's personal love, and in the saving power of his love.

4. Asking to be saved or to be healed, or that another person for whom you are praying be helped by the Lord; it is a good idea to ask explicitly, to describe in a prayer of petition the kind of help you are praying for.

5. Thanking and praising the Lord for his compassion, for the saving power of his love. This can take the form of praise and thanksgiving right away, in anticipation, as a form of trust in the Lord's response.

The psalms, including those of lament, have always been an important part of the church's worship (see Col 3:16; Eph 5:19), as they still are today. The psalms of lament make up part of the divine office, the official prayer of the church; and the Lamentations of Jeremiah are part of the Good Friday liturgy. The church herself laments, and teaches us to cry out to the Lord. We can call out to God in trust, because the risen Jesus stands *in the presence of God on our behalf* (Heb 9:24), *he always lives to make intercession for (us)* (Heb 7:25), praying the lament of the mediator. We can cry out to the Father in his name, and to Jesus himself who is our Savior.

Lord, have mercy on us.

Part II

THE CROSS AND INNER HEALING

FOUR

❧

By His Wounds We are Healed

THE CHRISTIAN TRADITION has always held that Jesus died not just for all people, but for each person as though that person were the only other person on earth. The mystery of the fact that God present in Jesus Christ loves each one of us personally, by name, without illusions and with total and unconditional acceptance, finds its center in the cross: that Jesus loves me so much as to have died to save me. No one can love more than to lay down his life for his friends; (cf. Jn 15:13). The cross weighs Jesus' love for me, tells me its measure.

This is one side of the equation, the cross as the measure of love; the other side is the power of that love to heal and to save, the power of Jesus' suffering and death, the healing power of his cross. Prayerfully entering into the healing structure of the cross of Jesus, we can enter more deeply into his love, and live better his wisdom — which is the foolishness of the cross.

*"We preach Christ crucified, a stumbling block to
the Jews and foolishness to the gentiles, but to those
who are the called, both Jews and Greeks, Christ,
the power of God and the wisdom of God. For God's
foolishness is wiser than human wisdom."*

1 COR 1:23 - 25

The Cross as Jesus' Experience of Sin

We can better understand the love of Jesus for each of us
through trying to understand better his experience, what
he underwent out of love for the Father and for his friends
— that is, for each of us.[1] To see the suffering of Jesus as
substitutionary, as vicarious suffering for our sins, does
not fully explain the mystery of the cross.[2] But it is a truth-
ful insight that Jesus *died for our sins* (1 Cor 15:3), that *he
gave his life as a ransom for many* (Mk 10:45), that *one man
died for the sake of the people* (cf. Jn 11:50). Jesus died for our
sins, that is, he suffered the consequences of sin, and so
experienced God's anger against him, the divine wrath
against all sinfulness. Jesus was so identified with sinners
that he, the Holy One became sin; *for our sake he (God) made
him to be sin who knew no sin* (2 Cor 5:21).

But is God really a God of anger? Does not Christianity
overcome the "just God" conception of the Old Testament
in Jesus' teaching about the loving mercy of our Father?
Marcion, the great second-century gnostic heretic,
thought so, and rejected the Old Testament's just God of
wrath for the New Testament's loving Father. The heresy
lay in thinking the two contradictory. They are not: *In God
there are mercy and wrath, support and pardon, but against the
impious he unleashes his anger* (Ecc/Sir 16:12). The Lord
strikes out against sinfulness, and — at the same time —
purifies and saves those who trust in him.

"Then he will speak to them in his wrath,
and terrify them in his anger . . .
Happy are those who take refuge in him."

PS 2:5, 11

" 'I will fulfill my words against this city for evil
and not for good . . .but I will deliver you on that
day,' says the Lord."

JER 39:16-17

The first chapter of Paul's Letter to the Romans teaches that God's anger is revealed through God's leaving those who persist in sin to the consequences of those same sins (vv.18-31) Sin contains the seed of its own punishment, and that punishment reveals the wrath of God against sin. The revelation of God's justice, the justice by which God justifies us, is revealed in the death of Jesus Christ,

". . . whom God put forward as an expiation by his
blood, to be received by faith. This was to show
God's righteousness, because in his divine
forbearance he had passed over former sins; it was
to prove at the present time that he himself is
righteous and that he justifies whoever has faith in
Jesus."

ROM 3:25-26

Through faith in Jesus Christ who died for us, we receive, in God's justice, forgiveness, justification. We have, then, nothing to fear from God's anger nor from his justice. In his anger against sin, he saves us from it, and in his justice, out of love for us, he saves us to himself; all this because Jesus Christ suffered and died for our sins.

"Where sin increased, grace abounded more, so that

grace might also exercise dominion through
justification leading to eternal life through Christ
our Lord."

ROM 5:21

Jesus' experience, then was one of *being made sin* for us, of carrying our sins and the *sin of the world*. He was without sin (Jn 8:46), but he was tried and tempted as we are, *one who, in every respect has been tempted as we are, yet without sin* (Heb 4:15). *He had to be made like his brethren in every respect . . . to make expiation for the sins of the people* (Heb 2:17-18). God, *sending his own Son in the likeness of sinful flesh and for sin, condemned sin in the flesh* (Rom 8:3). *For our sake, God made him to be sin who knew no sin, so that in him we might become the righteousness of God* (2 Cor 5:21).

Jesus' suffering and death expiate our sins. In the Bible, expiation is not the undergoing of punishment for sin, nor is it the mere appeasement of an angry God by an act of sacrifice. Primarily, expiation means the annihilation of sin, the destruction of sin, by a sacrificial act. "Expiation does not act upon God himself, but upon the sinner inasmuch as it purifies him from sin."[3] Dying, Jesus triumphs over death and so over sin and its consequences, for *the sting of sin is death; 'O death, where is your sting?'* (1 Cor 15: 56a, 55b).

None of this means anything, of course, if we fail to understand the cross as an act of love, both on the part of the Father who sent his only Son to save us, and on Jesus' part, who lays down his life in love. Jesus' expiation is done for love and in love: *In this is love, not that we loved God but that he loved us and sent his Son to be the expiation for our sins* (1 Jn 4:10).

"If God is for us, who is against us? He who did
not spare his own Son but gave him up for us all,

> *will he not also give us all things with him? . . .*
> *Who can separate us from the love of Christ? . . .*
> *We are more than conquerors through him who*
> *loved us. For I am sure that neither death, nor life,*
> *nor angels, nor principalities, nor things present,*
> *nor things to come, nor powers, nor height, nor*
> *depth, nor anything else in all creation, can sepa-*
> *rate us from the love of God in Christ Jesus our*
> *Lord."*

ROM 8:31-39

This said, let us examine the gospels to try to enter into the interior experience of Jesus, his psychological experience, what he felt.

Jesus' Psychological Experience of the Cross

Jesus foresaw and even predicted his own suffering and death. He accepted the brutal torture and ugly death without flinching, though not without an agonizing struggle as he prayed in the garden, and, above all, with his eyes open, not denying to himself or others what the future held. He had realized what lay ahead in Jerusalem: *"I have a baptism with which to be baptized, and what stress I am under until it is completed!"* (Lk 12:50). Jesus might well have made his own the words of Isaiah:

> *"The Lord God helps me;*
> *therefore I have not been disgraced;*
> *I have set my face like flint,*
> *and I know that I will not be put to shame;*
> *he who vindicates me is close by."*

IS 50:7-8

*"He began to teach them that the Son of man must
suffer many things, and be rejected by the chief
priests and the scribes, and be killed, and after three
days rise again. But Peter took him, and began to
rebuke him."*

MK 8:31-33

Jesus' answering rebuke to Peter, *"Get behind me Satan;
for you are not on the side of God, but of men"* (Mk 8:33),
expresses Jesus' resistance to the temptation to deny the
reality of what is coming. He rejects, strongly, the temptation; and he encourages his followers to have that same
clear-minded realism and to take up the cross and follow
him (8:34-38). He predicts his passion again (9:30-32), and
a third time, describing in more detail what will happen:
his condemnation to death in Jerusalem, where they are
headed; his consignment to the Roman forces of occupa-
tion; the mocking and the scourging (10:32-3). He foretells
Judas' betrayal and Peter's denial, accepting both with
resignation and a certain calm (14:18,30).

In the context of his imminent torture and death, his
anger against the kind of sinful blindness and crassness
that is to crucify him appears as natural, normal, and certainly understandable. We recognize Jesus' unusual
behavior in violently driving the buyers and sellers out of
the Temple as normal, not as deviant conduct; the Temple
is being profaned just as the new temple, his own body,
will very soon be profaned and hideously mistreated (Mk
11:15-18). Luke situates the cleaning out of the Temple just
after Jesus' messianic entry into Jerusalem, as do Mark
and Matthew, and immediately after his weeping over
Jerusalem, so high-lighting the pathos of his anger. In the
light of the cross, Jesus' anger against the blind hypocrisy
and resistance of the leaders of Israel can be seen as anger

against that very sinfulness and darkness whose hour is coming shortly on Calvary.

Jesus knows what Israel's religious leaders are plotting against him, but he does not give in at all. He does not try to make a bargain. This uncompromising fidelity to the truth he proclaims, and to the Father's loving will continues throughout the last supper and the passion. Before Annas and Caiaphas, Jesus does not defend himself, does not bargain. He stands silent in front of Herod, and does no miracle or feat that might help his cause. (Pilate sent Jesus captive, to Herod: *Herod was very glad, for he had been wanting to see him for a long time, because he had heard about him and was hoping to see him perform some sign* (Lk 23:7-8). He refuses to negotiate with Pilate. What seems in all this, to be stoicism is really the refusal of the temptation to bargain or to negotiate in the face of his suffering and death.

In the agony in the garden of Gethsemane, this same inner strength crumbles and dissolves, leaving only its source: adhesion to the Father's will. It reappears after Jesus' prayer in the garden as he rises from prayer and meets the armed men who have come to take him prisoner. What happened in Jesus' agony in the garden of Gethsemane? What did Jesus experience there? He describes it himself: *"My soul is in anguish, even to death"* (Mk 14:34); he is *greatly distressed and troubled* (Mk 14:33). In other words, Jesus suffers not only fear, but severe depression. Luke's gospel describes Jesus' condition with the sentence: *and being in agony, he prayed more earnestly; and his sweat became like great drops of blood falling down upon the ground* (Lk 22:44). Sweating blood, perspiring mixed water and blood, is a symptom of a total physical and psychological breakdown, of an extremely grave depression which would be expected to end in death.

And yet, Jesus somehow works through that severe

depression in his prayer in Gethsemane. His interior resistance and revulsion to the passion and to death (for Jesus *is* Life: *'I am . . . life'* (Jn 11:25), lead him to cry out: *"Abba, Father, all things are possible to you; remove this cup from me"* (Mk 14:36a). The prospect of drinking the cup of God's anger, of the divine wrath and judgment against sin, forces Jesus into a complete breakdown, into a severe depression. In agony of mind he continues to pray: *"Not my will, but yours be done"* (Mk 14:36b). Centering himself and his prayer on this — that the Father's will be done — Jesus pulls himself together enough to warn his sleeping companions, Peter, James and John, and to be prepared to meet the men coming to arrest him: *"Get up, let us be going. Look, my betrayer is here"* (Mk 14:42).

The fruit of this suffering and of this acceptance of the Father's will is a compassion so great as to be nearly unbelievable. Jesus' first act after his agony is to heal the ear of the slave of the high priest (Lk 22:51). Then he gives himself up, protecting his disciples: *"I am he. So if you are looking for me, let these men go"* (Jn 18:8). Nailed to the cross, he forgives the very people who are murdering him, praying that the Father forgive them, and even excusing them in his prayer (Lk 23:34). One of the thieves crucified with him asks to be remembered; Jesus forgives him and promises him Paradise that same day (Lk 23:42-43). He shows compassion to his mother, putting her in the care of John (Jn 19:26-27).

Shortly before Jesus dies, he cries out to the Father: *"My God, my God, why have you abandoned me?"* (Mk 15:34). God feels abandoned by God; Life is dying. Practically incapable of prayer, laden with the hideous sins of the world, in physical and mental torment, he cries out in lament to his Father. God is dying, abandoned by God. At his baptism in the river Jordan, Jesus had heard his Father's

voice: *"You are my beloved Son; in you I delight"* (Lk 3:22).
Now there is only the mocking echo from his tormentors:
"He trusts in God; let God deliver him now if he wants to" (Mt
27:43). And they taunt him with the very Psalm he is trying to pray: *"let him rescue him, the one in whom he delights"*
(Ps 22:8). There is no answer from heaven. His Father has
turned his face away. That death is an act of love by Jesus
for us and for the Father; and the Father gives Jesus up to
death in an act of love for us and for Jesus. Their love for
one another here becomes radical sacrifice. And that
mutual love is the Holy Spirit, whose name is Love, and
who is poured into our hearts by Jesus and his Father.
Love gives meaning to the sacrifice.

Finally, Jesus gives a loud cry: *"Father, into your hands I
commend my spirit,"* and dies (Lk 23:46). Feeling completely abandoned, he abandons himself in death to his Father
in an act of supreme, unfelt, trust. The prayer *"into your
hands I commend my spirit"* is from a psalm of lament,
Psalm 31:5. It probably formed a part of a common Jewish
death-bed prayer.[4]

John's gospel reports two other exclamations of Jesus in
his dying moments. Knowing that all is finished, Jesus
says, *"I thirst;"* as he dies, he says, *"It is finished"* (19:28,30).
Surely Jesus suffered from physical thirst. But John wants
us to understand Jesus' thirst also in a spiritual sense; his
thirst is his desire to give the living water of the Spirit.[5]
The coming of the Spirit depends on Jesus' dying, and in
giving up his spirit Jesus communicates to us, gives, his
Spirit. This is the meaning of the blood and water that
issue from the dead Jesus' side when it is pierced by the
soldier's spear. The blood is the blood of Jesus' sacrifice; it
symbolizes his life-giving redemptive love. The water
symbolizes the Holy Spirit, the fountain of living water
(see Jn 7:37-39; Zec 12:10; 13:1). The water mixed with

blood prefigures the permanent outpouring of the Spirit after Jesus' death.[6] And Jesus' Spirit is the Spirit of healing.

The Power of the Cross to Heal

It is easy to think of Jesus' suffering and death as punishment for sin, but this would be an error. God is not sadistic, and suffering is not a punishment he administers for sinning. Refusing God's love, separating from him, turning away from him — and these are what sin is — is its own punishment. Holding suffering to be punishment for sin, sometimes masks an attitude of contempt toward the afflicted; they are viewed as suffering because they are sinners. *"Rabbi, who sinned, this man or his parents?"* asked the disciples about the man blind from birth. Jesus' reply is firm: *"Neither this man nor his parents sinned"* (Jn 9:1). The attitude of the Father and of Jesus — they have the same attitude, for Jesus is the revelation of the Father — is just the opposite of contempt. It is compassion. Jesus, crucified outside the walls of the city, finds himself — rather chooses to be — identified with those outside the *cives*, outside civility and civilization — the outcasts, the forgotten, the despised, the hopelessly marginal and those beyond all margin. He suffers the treatment not of a common criminal but, worse, of an uncommon criminal, the charges trumped up, his trial a travesty, his torture brutally evil, and his execution a horror. And he takes upon himself the neediness of the abandoned, the poor, the oppressed, the agonizing, and of all of us in whatever way we are consciously or unconsciously needy. He identifies with those who need to be saved so as to save them. He is "made sin" for sinners. He becomes one with all of us who need healing so that we may be healed.

He was crucified in weakness (2 Cor 13:4) so that we can *glory in our own weakness and that the power of Christ may rest upon us; for when we are weak, we are strong* (2 Cor 12:9). *God chose what is weak in the world to shame the strong* (1 Cor 1:27), *for the weakness of God is stronger than men* (1 Cor 1:25). God's power is made perfect in the weakness of Jesus crucified; it is through the power of the cross that the Father has chosen to reconcile all things to himself in Jesus Christ (Eph 2:16; Col 1:20), to knot things together making them whole, unifying and healing. Paul also proclaims the power of the cross, and the cross as the power of God (1 Cor 1:17-18). This is not to take away from the power of the resurrection, but to say that for Paul "the resurrection in fact begins at the moment of [Jesus'] death: . . . people are converted, the centurion confesses the faith, the Holy Spirit is poured out."[7]

For John's gospel, too, Jesus' death rather than his resurrection is the completion of his work because by the cross the sources of eternal life are open to us. The cross has the power to save.

John's gospel proclaims the healing power of the cross by comparing it with the bronze serpent that Moses, following God's instructions, placed on a pole (Num 21:4-9). Those who had been bitten by snakes looked at the serpent and were healed. *Just as Moses lifted up the serpent in the wilderness, so must the Son of man be lifted up that whoever believes may have eternal life in him* (Jn 3:14-15). And so John quotes Zechariah in reference to Jesus' side being opened by the spear: *They shall look on him whom they have pierced* (Jn 19:37; Zec 12:10).

In the act of saving us, Jesus is mocked; the gospel writers do not want us to miss the irony of this mockery, unintentional irony for the mockers, but consciously included in the gospel.

*"And those who passed by made fun of him,
wagging their heads and saying, 'Aha! You who
would destroy the temple and build it in three days,
save yourself, and come down from the cross!' So
also the chief priests mocked him to one another
with the scribes, saying, 'He saved others; he
cannot save himself . . .'"*

MK 15:31

There is a double irony. The religious leaders give testimony to Jesus' healings through their mocking words. He *saved others* could have no other meaning than that Jesus healed sicknesses, cast out demons, raised the dead to life. Secondly, they make fun of Jesus for his weakness in the very hour that the power of God in Jesus saves the world. The saving and healing power of God cannot be dissociated from the cross of Jesus. Dennis Hamm has put the point concisely:

> The healing ministry of Jesus is fully
> understood only in the context of the saving
> death of Jesus. This is the clear message of the
> evangelists. Matthew, Mark and Luke, in their
> descriptions of the crucifixion, present Jesus as
> the hanged leader. Jesus is taunted, "He saved
> others; he cannot save himself." The reference
> is, of course, to the healing ministry. And the
> evangelist includes the taunt, one suspects,
> because of the profound irony the words carry
> for the Christian reader: the hanged healer
> does indeed heal and save most deeply
> through his saving death. Luke underscores
> this in his version of the second passion
> prediction (Lk 9:43b-44): But while they were
> all marvelling at everything he did (the

healing of the demoniac has just been
narrated), he said to his disciples, "Let these
words sink into your ears, for the son of man
is to be delivered into the hands of men." In
other words, the appreciation of Jesus' healing
ministry is not to be separated from the
meaning of his passion and death.[8]

And it is the Christian tradition from the beginning,
that by Jesus' wounds we are healed. The fourth song of
Deutero Isaiah's Suffering Servant prophesies this:

*"He was despised, the lowest of men: a man of
pains, familiar with disease, One from whom men
turn away; despised, and we reckoned him as
nothing. But he took our sickness away, he carried
away our diseases. While we counted him as one
struck down, afflicted by God. He was wounded for
our rebelliousness, crushed for our sins; The
punishment that has reconciled us fell upon him,
and by his wounds we are healed."*

IS 53:3-5[9]

Matthew's gospel sees the healings of Jesus' public ministry as fulfilling the Suffering Servant prophecy: ". . . *he
cast out the spirits with a word, and healed all who were sick.
This was to fulfill what was spoken by the prophet Isaiah, 'He
took our sickness; carried away our diseases'."* (Mt 8:16b-17).
Peter's First Letter makes the application to the passion
and death of Jesus: *He himself bore our sins in his body on the
tree, so that we might die to sin and live to righteousness. By his
wounds you have been healed* (2:24).

We can be healed simply by looking at Jesus, by looking upon *him whom they have pierced,* just as the Hebrews
looked upon the raised metal serpent and were healed.
Also we can pray for healing by prayerfully taking our

own wounds into the structure of Jesus' passion and death. This is the purpose of the next chapter.

🍃

FIVE

The Cross and Prayer for Inner Healing

THE CROSS is a statement to us, a "word" about God and about ourselves; it reveals God, and in his light we too are revealed. The word of the cross reveals its power, the power made perfect in the weakness of the Crucified. Because the word of the cross speaks God's power in weakness, it is a word of wisdom that appears as foolishness (see 1 Cor 1:18-25).

The Foolishness of the Cross

To proclaim the cross appears foolish. Further, how could anyone be healed through the cross? To speak of the healing *power* of the cross seems a contradiction, for the cross at first glance means *weakness*. In the eyes of the world, the cross seems more than foolish, it appears as folly, as lunacy.

The Old Testament has a tradition of the wisdom of the

wise seen by God as foolishness. The wisdom of Egypt appears at the Exodus as stupidity: *The princes of Zoan are utterly foolish; the wise counselors of Pharaoh give stupid counsel* (Is 19:11a). Isaiah deplores those who think themselves wise, but who call good "evil," and evil "good": *"Woe to those who are wise in their own eyes"* (5:21), as does Jeremiah: *"The wise men shall be put to shame, they shall be dismayed and taken; lo, they have rejected the word of the Lord, and what wisdom is in them?"* (8:9). God's wisdom is infinitely above ours, beyond our logic:

> *"For my thoughts are not your thoughts,*
> *my ways are not your ways, says the Lord.*
> *As the heavens are higher than the earth,*
> *so are my ways higher than your ways and*
> *my thoughts above your thoughts."*

IS 55:8-9

God's wisdom so far transcends ours that it can appear to us as foolishness. Job, unable to understand his miserable condition, complains loudly; the wisdom of his friends does not give him an answer. The Lord says, *"Shall a faultfinder contend with the Almighty?"* and Job puts his hand over his mouth and remains silent in face of what is so far above him that it seems completely unreasonable (Jb 40: 2-3). The human view is partial; it cannot know everything; *even though a wise man claims to know, he cannot find it out* (Ecc 8:17b).

> *"The kings of the earth set themselves, and the*
> *rulers take counsel together, against the*
> *Lord and his anointed . . .*
> *He who sits in the heavens laughs; the Lord*
> *mocks them . . .*
> *Now therefore, O kings, be wise . . .*

Serve the Lord with fear, with trembling."

PS 2:2-11

For Paul, the cross marks the definitive triumph of God's wisdom; the words of Isaiah, *"I will destroy the wisdom of the wise, and the cleverness of the clever I will bring to nothing,"* come true in a radical way in the suffering and death of Jesus, in the triumph of the cross (1 Cor 1:19; referring to Is 29:14). By the cross, *God has made foolish the wisdom of this world* (1 Cor 1:20b); and so *the world's wisdom is foolishness to God* (1 Cor 3:19a). Because of the foolishness of the cross, Paul becomes *a fool for Christ's sake* (1 Cor 4:10).

So too, in praying for inner healing, an attitude of "being a fool for Christ" is a help. The qualities that go with being a fool — simplicity, openness, complete trust — make one more receptive to God's healing power. At the same time, inner healing is not a matter of scientific or psychological wisdom, not of self-knowledge; it is a matter of grace, of *the love of God poured into our hearts through the Holy Spirit,* a love that heals us. The wisdom of God transcends human wisdom, goes so far beyond it as to look like lunacy, and so far that human wisdom itself is, by comparison, foolishness. The power of the inner healing that comes through prayer goes way beyond the power of psychology and of every merely human approach. It is a question of going to the Lord like a child, or like a fool, simply, and asking for healing. One way to do this is to put our own hurts into the context of the cross of Jesus so that they may be healed. Saint Bonaventure has written:

> The cross is our book, in which is written the whole wisdom of Christ . . . Only the cross can free you . . . The best thing to meditate on is the cross . . . So we should take up the cross of

Christ as a book of wisdom, in which we see ourselves.[1]

Looking *on him whom they have pierced*, I can see his love for me, and — at the same time, in his light — see myself with my interior hurts, my weakness, my neediness. This "looking" can free me, heal me, make me more whole.

Praying about Our Hurts in the Light of Jesus' Passion

The previous chapter described Jesus' psychological experience of his passion in eight steps:

1. Jesus foresaw his coming passion and death, and accepted it with open eyes.

2. Anger appears in his reaction, anger against the abuse of the Temple (a symbol of his body), and anger against the religious leaders who are plotting his murder.

3. He rejects the temptation to bargain with those who will kill him, just as later he refuses to negotiate with Annas, Caiaphas, Herod and Pilate.

4. He undergoes deathly depression in the garden of Gethsemane.

5. He embraces the Father's will, accepting his death, its form, and the suffering leading up to it.

These five steps lead up to Jesus' death. The next three represent the psychological phases he passes through in his dying on the cross.

6. Compassion: he forgives his killers and the thief, and speaks compassionately to his mother and to John.

7. Feeling abandoned: *My God, my God, why have you forsaken me?*

8. Delivering himself into the Father's hands in death so that the new age of the outpouring of the Spirit can

begin.

The last three psychological phases, the interior states of Jesus' dying, are marked by the "seven last words", three of compassion, one of abandonment, and three of consigning himself to the Father in a new beginning for the world. The first five steps follow the five stages of dying described by Elizabeth Kubler-Ross in *On Death and Dying*.[2] Dr Kubler-Ross describes how terminally ill patients typically go through five psychological stages as death approaches:

1. denial of the fact that they are dying
2. anger that this is happening to them
3. bargaining with the doctor or with God to save them from dying
4. depression
5. acceptance of death

Jesus was like us in everything except sin, so it comes as unsurprising that he suffered through the typical process of those close to death.

Matthew and Dennis Linn, in their book *Healing Life's Hurts*, pray through Elizabeth Kubler-Ross's five stages of dying "so that the crippling hurts of life become opportunities for emotional, physical, and spiritual healing."[3] We can adapt the ideas of the Linn brothers to apply them in a prayer that works through the stages of Jesus' psychological experience, entering into his experiences as well as we can, placing our own painful memories and hurtful experiences in his so that by his wounds we may be healed.[4] We will pray through not only the five Kubler-Ross stages, which the Linns have adapted to prayer for inner healing, but also through the three stages of Jesus' dying on the cross.

Each of us has one or more crosses to carry. It might be a cross connected with work; it could be a person or a few people who, wittingly, or unwittingly, make life difficult for me; it could be an illness, or a physical or emotional handicap; it could be a pattern of sin that resists being done away with. It could be something I carry from the past: a memory that needs healing; past failure or disgrace; an unhappy childhood; a loss through death. I can ask the Lord to guide me as to what cross to carry, in prayer, in union with his suffering, so that his wounds may heal mine.

Taking Up the Cross and Following Jesus in Prayer

"If anyone would come after me, let him deny himself and take up his cross and follow me" (Mk 8:34b). I can deny myself the luxury of self-pity and of hanging on to resentment or hurt, and I can take up my particular cross, in prayer, with Jesus.

1. Facing reality

    Lord Jesus, help me to face my cross squarely. You were completely realistic in facing yours; give me the grace of sharing in that realism. Let me see my cross, my situation as you see it, through your eyes. Thank you for the growth involved, for whatever is good in the situation. I ask you to strengthen me to see my own hurt with my eyes open, not denying any of the more painful aspects.

(At this point I can describe the situation to the Lord in my own words, speaking as to a friend who understands perfectly.)

2. Working through resentment and anger

    Lord, help me to recognize any anger in myself about this situation. You were not afraid of being

*angry; help me to recognize and to feel the anger or
rage or resentment or bitterness or sullenness
inside me. I unite that anger to the anger that you
felt during your last time in Jerusalem, knowing
how it would end. Show me what anger lies inside
me, and against whom. Show me where I am hurt
and what was and is the reaction in me to that hurt
and to what hurt me or continues to hurt me.*

(Describe the hurt and your reaction to it to the Lord,
using any emotional language that comes to mind, "getting out to him" any resentment, anger, hostility, and the
roots of any coldness or defensiveness in you).

*Take out of my heart, Lord, any anger or
resentment that is not from you, that blocks me
from forgiving and from loving. I give you this
hostility; take it, Lord; fill me that I may be free to
love. Take away my resentful defensiveness, my
hardness of heart, and give me a heart of flesh, a
compassionate heart like yours.*

3. Resisting the temptation to bargain

*Lord, you accepted your suffering without trying
futilely to change those who made you suffer,
without making conditions or demanding that
things be different. Teach me and help me to be like
you, to accept what I cannot change, and to carry
the cross of what I cannot change in union with
you.*

(Take a moment to look at the Lord and to let him show
you whether you are putting conditions on your suffering,
such as demanding that other people or the situation be

different. Speak to him in your own words.)

4. Working through sadness and depression

*Lord, through your own sadness unto death in
your agony in the garden, heal me of all sadness or
depression and darkness of mind. Help me to
recognize any fear or dread in myself, and any grief
or sadness. Fill me with your love that casts out all
fear and despondency and every spirit of
depression. By your emotional wounds in the
garden of Gethsemane, heal my emotional wounds,
and fill the healed places with your love and
unconditional acceptance of me just as I am now.*

(Let the Lord heal you of any depression — which can
be anger turned in against yourself, self-hatred — by filling you with his personal love for you. Give him any fear
you have, and let him take it away. Tell him how you feel
about this cross, and accept his healing power.)

5. Acceptance of the cross

*Lord Jesus, I accept this cross, and with you I say
to the Father: "Father, all things are possible to
you; remove this cup from me; however, not my
will, but yours be done." Help me to see the
possibilities of growth in this cross; you write
straight with crooked lines; show me the positive
side of this cross. I accept it for love of you, in
union with you and accepting your compassionate
love for me.*

(Tell the Lord that, with his strength, you embrace this
cross for him and with him, as your response to his love
of you.)

Heal me, Lord, so that I can not only accept this

cross, but also praise you for everything, including the negative things in my life.

Praying with Jesus Crucified

Paul writes, *"I have been crucified with Christ; it is no longer I who live, but Christ who lives in me"* (Gal 2:20). You can continue to pray about the cross in your life, looking at Jesus on the cross and drawing strength from the healing power of the Crucified. The answer to the song's question, "Were you there when they crucified my Lord?" is "I am there now in prayer."

6. Forgiving

Lord, you can forgive your murderers and pray for them. Forgive me. And give me the power of your forgiveness on the cross so that I can forgive those who have hurt and those who have wronged me. I trust in the power to forgive that you have and that you give me. And before you now, I forgive all who have hurt me.

(Forgive each person who has knowingly or unknowingly contributed to the cross you are praying about. Tell the Lord that you forgive each one, mentioning the person by name and praying for that person.)

Give me, Lord, a compassionate and forgiving heart towards each person who has hurt me.

7. Crying out to the Lord

Lord, I cry out to you. Sometimes I feel alone and abandoned, and you seem far away. Out of the depths I cry to you, Lord.

(Do not hesitate truly to lament to the Lord. You might use one of the psalms of lament, such as Psalm 22 or Psalm 69.)

8. Abandonment to the Lord

Lord Jesus Christ, I abandon myself completely to you. With you, I cry out to our Father, "Father, into your hands I commend my spirit." And Lord, like you in your suffering and death, I thirst. I thirst for a new outpouring of your healing Spirit of love on me and on those dear to me. Come, Lord Jesus.

Praying in Other Ways for Healing through the Cross

Christian tradition has developed ways of praying through the suffering and death of Jesus, ways that many find helpful more than ever today, for example, the Eucharist, the stations of the cross, devotion to the heart of Jesus, the *Spiritual Exercises* of Ignatius Loyola, and praying through the sorrowful mysteries of the rosary. Unfortunately, these ways of praying sometimes seem to be followed with little or no thought of the healing power of Jesus, and in his loving willingness to heal us. Nevertheless, they remain valuable ways of contemplating the Lord's passion, especially when prayed with faith and trust that in Jesus' suffering and death we find healing and salvation.

Sometimes our sorrow or grief or hurt is beyond expression in words. The psalmist experienced this:

*"Because my heart was made bitter
and my soul was pierced,
I was stupid and did not understand;*

I was like a dumb animal in your presence.
Yet with you I will always be;
you hold my right hand."

PS 73:21-23

That prayer of pain is one Jesus on the cross knew all about. We can take the advice of the anonymous four-teenth century author of *The Book of Privy Counseling:*

> Do as I tell you now, he says, Take the good
> gracious God just as he is, as plain as a
> common poultice, and lay him to your sick
> self, just as you are. Or, if I may put it another
> way, lift up your sick self, just as you are, and
> let your desire reach out to touch the good,
> gracious God, just as he is, for to touch him is
> eternal health.[5]

The celebration of the Eucharist, the way *par excellence* to pray about the Lord's passion and death, commemo-rates the Last Supper; since the Last Supper anticipated the sacrifice of the cross, every Eucharist re-presents not only the Lord's supper but also his sacrificial death. The Eucharist applies the healing power of the cross of Jesus.[6]

Matthew and Dennis Linn give valuable suggestions for praying the Stations of the Cross for the healing of memories, with a prayer outline; they suggest:

> One memory of a hurt can be handled in
> greater depth by watching Christ in each
> station deal with what I felt when hurt. Thus
> the memory of being humiliated during
> seventh grade while giving a wrong answer
> on TV can be healed as I watch Christ dealing
> with humiliation in each station. The process is

one of giving Christ my feelings and taking on
his reactions.[7]

The fourteen Stations of the Cross (the "Way of the
Cross") can be found along the side walls of most Catholic
churches and chapels, but they can be followed anywhere,
praying through them silently, perhaps using a New
Testament account of the passion.[8]

Another part of Christian tradition skips the historical
details and goes right to the heart of Jesus' motivation in
his passion, his love. In particular, devotion to the heart of
Jesus, pierced by the spear, underlines the love of Jesus for
each person; the heart symbolizes Jesus' love. Catherine of
Siena sums up the Christian life in terms of love and
union with Jesus crucified: "You will find the source of
love in the side of Christ crucified, and that is where I
wish you to seek your refuge and your abode."[9] Julian of
Norwich, describing her prayer, writes:

> He led my understanding to this same wound
> in his side. And there, within, he showed a fair
> and delightful place, large enough for all
> mankind that shall be saved, to rest there, in
> peace and in love. Herewith he brought to my
> mind the most dear and precious water which
> he let pour out for love . . . Forthwith this
> good Lord said most blissfully, "See, how I
> have loved you."[10]

The wisdom of the *Spiritual Exercises* of Ignatius Loyola
is the foolishness of the cross,[11] and instructive for prayer
for healing through the cross. Ignatius advises the use of
the imagination: "Imagine Christ our Lord present before
you on the cross . . . As I behold Christ in this plight, I shall
ponder what presents itself to my mind."[12] Even more

often, he advises bringing the emotions into play. Praying about the passion, we are advised to ask for "sorrow, compassion, and shame, because the Lord is going to his sufferings for my sins,"[13] for "sorrow with Christ in sorrow, anguish with Christ in anguish, tears and deep grief because of the great affliction Christ endures for me."[14] Notice that these feelings are God's gift, graces of prayer, that we are to ask for. Yet, at the same time, Ignatius counsels us to co-operate with these graces and even to anticipate them, "to make a great effort . . . to be sad and grieve because of the great sorrow and suffering of Christ the Lord."[15] And again, "I will rouse myself to sorrow, suffering and anguish by frequently calling to mind the labors, fatigue, and suffering which Christ our Lord endured from the time of his birth down to the mystery of the passion upon which I am engaged at present."[16]

Ignatius focuses not so much on the material aspects of Jesus' suffering as on the interior attitudes. We are asked to contemplate "what Christ suffers in his human nature," "what he desires to suffer," the most sacred humanity suffering so cruelly," "that Christ suffers all this for my sins," "the great fear that overwhelmed him."[17] Ignatius emphasizes the death of Jesus "for my sins" and "for me." He stresses Jesus as *my* Savior. "I am the meaning of Christ's cross."[18] It measures his love for me. And Jesus calls me to share in his sufferings, to enter into his experience, to suffer and to anguish with him. "It is only by actually experiencing, with God's grace and in my own way, what he experiences that I will also experience how he has transformed this dying experience into a new creation."[19] And so through my own dying experience now or in the past, through my own cross, I can be healed into a new creation.

Ignatius also suggests contemplating "the presence" at the cross "of his most sorrowful mother," "her great sorrow and weariness, and also that of the disciples."[20] This leads to the role of Mary, the mother of Jesus, in praying for healing through the cross.

SIX

Jesus' Mother at the Cross

"All you who pass by, look and see
if there is any sorrow like my sorrow."

LAM 1:12

MARY THE MOTHER OF JESUS was no stranger to sorrow and suffering. From the visit of the angel at Nazareth, her troubles began — pregnant before she and Joseph *had come together* (Mt 1:18), so that Joseph was planning *to put her away privately.* No doubt she lost her reputation as the quick eyes and tongues of the other women were at work. Then the child is born, in an unsanitary stable, with animal smells and dung. Soon after comes the shock of Simeon's dark prophesy, turning a happy day of the child's presentation in the Temple, to a foreboding that was to follow her all her life: *"This child is destined . . . to be a sign that will be opposed . . . and a sword will pierce you own soul too"* (Lk 2:34-35). At each crisis, Mary must have thought the time had come for harm to her child. Soon Herod *is about to search for the child* (Mt 2:13), and the young family become political refugees from the massacre they escape. Then in Egypt they live as immigrants, foreigners, desperate for a house and for work, open to the discrimination that immigrants attract. After Herod's death they return to the ordinary life of Nazareth, until the nightmare three days when they lose the child in Jerusalem. The fear, self reproach, dread of those days is known to many parents with a missing child.

After the quiet years when they returned to Nazareth and Jesus grew up, came his public life, and the immediate confrontation with the authorities. Mary must have seen where things were headed; must have known the inevitable outcome. She saw on the road to Calvary what had been done to him. Her son, to her *the most beautiful of the sons of men* (Ps 45:3) had become:

> *"a man of suffering,*
> *accustomed to infirmity,*
> *One of those from whom men*
> *turn away."*

IS 53:3

The sorrows of Mary are traditionally remembered as the Seven Dolors, or Sorrows. One can pray them as a rosary of seven decades of seven beads, or meditate — be with Mary in contemplating her great sorrow. The Seven Dolors are:

1. The presentation of the child Jesus in the Temple
2. The flight into Egypt
3. The loss of the boy Jesus in Jerusalem
4. Mary meets her son on the road to Calvary
5. Mary stands at the foot of the cross
6. Jesus is taken down from the cross and laid in his mother's arms
7. Jesus is buried.

In that meeting on the road, and standing at the cross,

Mary knew that Jesus was dying for her as for us. She is a creature as we are, and so needed his saving death. True she never sinned, and because of the foreseen merits of her son, she was conceived without the weakness of original sin. Yet her human feelings must have included anger like Jesus' own anger. And did heaven seem shut to her as it was to Jesus? *"Though I call and cry for help, he (God) shuts out my prayer"* (Lam 3:8). Sharing Jesus' agony in her heart, she said "Yes" to the Father, in utter abandonment, even to the giving, like the Father, of her only son. *Jesus Christ,* Paul tells us (2 Cor 1:19) *was not "Yes" and "No;" but in him it is always "Yes."* And so with Mary, from that first "Yes," the *fiat* at Nazareth. *"Be it done to me according to your word"* (Lk 1:38) is an echo of Jesus': *"Father, not my will but yours"* (Lk 22:42).

Then Jesus, looking down on his mother asks her to take us, in the person of John, as her children. This is in the moment when the sin of the world is crucifying him. Utter forgiveness of us is her response,

> Mary, in a miracle of love, so that she might receive us as her children, offered generously to the Divine Justice her own Son, and in her heart died with him, stabbed by the sword of sorrow.
>
> POPE LEO XIII[1]

How could Mary ever be healed interiorly of such suffering? *Vast as the sea is your ruin; who can heal you?* (Lam 2:13). Jesus was healed in the resurrection, but it is significant that he kept the marks of the wounds in his hands and side. Inner healing is not the taking away of wounds, but of taking away the negativity, and of making the healed places strong and even glorious. Wherever our blessed Lady has appeared on earth, Lourdes, Fatima, etc.

always there are healings — physical and inner, in fact there is never a physical healing without an inner, even more wonderful transformation. We can go to Mary for inner healing of the most unbearable sufferings, the loss of a child, of a spouse — especially if caused by negligence or malice of others. Nothing, great or small is outside her compassion.

Luke's gospel understands Mary as a model for the Christian and also as a figure of the faithful remnant of Israel, of the "poor" who remain faithful to God through suffering (Lk 1:48,52; Zep 2:3; 3:12-15). Luke associates Mary with Jesus' redemptive suffering as Simeon prophesies: *"This child is set . . . for a sign that is spoken against; and a sword will pierce through your own heart also"* (Lk 2:34b-35a). But it is John's gospel that describes Mary's place at the foot of the cross.

For John, Mary is principally a model of faith. Her faith at the cross continues the faith she showed at the wedding party of Cana (Jn 2:1-12). John's gospel puts Cana and the cross in parallel. They mark the beginning and end of Jesus' public ministry; in both, Mary is referred to as Jesus' mother, and called by Jesus "woman;" and both texts refer to a providential "hour." John clearly intends these three parallels to symbolize deeper realities.

At Cana, Mary asks Jesus to work a miracle in order to save the embarrassment of the hosts for running out of wine. At her asking, he does it. In keeping with the spirit of John's own gospel, I can ask Mary to do what she did at Cana: ask Jesus to save the situation. I can ask anyone to pray for me or with me, or both; so too, with greater reason because of the precedent of Cana, can I ask Jesus' mother to pray with me and for me for the inner healing that comes from the power of Jesus' cross.[2] She is his mother, and she was there at his death.

Furthermore, Mary is my mother. Besides my biological

mother, and perhaps someone else who took her role in bringing me up, I have a mother in heaven who is Jesus' own mother.

Jesus came to us first, in the Incarnation, and in his birth, through Mary. That is, Mary is his mother. "is," not "was his mother." Because motherhood is a permanent relationship. Your mother is always, permanently, your mother, and always will be. Because Mary's motherhood is a permanent relationship, because Jesus came to us first at the beginning of that relationship, because he came to us first through Mary, he comes to us always through Mary. The life of Jesus in me, the life of grace, comes to me through Mary. This is what the doctrine of Mary as Mediatrix of grace means. All graces come from the Father in Jesus through the Holy Spirit; and they come through God's door to the human world: Mary.

This descending mediation of grace does not necessarily imply the need for ascending mediation. That grace comes through Mary does not at all mean that I must go through her to get it. I can pray directly to Jesus. I can pray directly to the Father.

Descending mediation means that ascending mediation is possible. I *can* ask Mary to pray for me. In that sense, I can pray to her.

She is my mother in the spiritual order because she is the mother of the life of Jesus in me, the Mediatrix of grace. Jesus himself ratified this personal spiritual motherhood of Mary for each of us just before his death on the cross.

He said to Mary his mother standing with John the apostle at the foot of the cross, *"Woman, this is your child."* Then Jesus spoke to John, saying, *"This is your mother"* (Jn 19:26-27). Christian tradition has always held that John was standing in for each one of us as he stood at the cross near the mother of Jesus. Jesus gave you to his mother when he died on the cross. And he gave his own mother to you as your mother.

Since Mary is my mother, I can pray to her for inner healing. I can ask her to pray for me to Jesus for interior healing. And I can pray with Mary, go with her to God to pray for healing.

Praying for inner healing, I can cry out to God with her, lamenting with her.[3] I can join my lament to her sorrow at the foot of the cross, joining my hurts to hers. I can pray to the Father, with Jesus' mother:

> Times and seasons change
> centuries and ages pass;
> you seem above them, Lord,
> untouched, unmoved.
>
> But
> your Son entered in,
> born of a woman,
> crushed and crucified,
> to ransom us.
>
> Will you be deaf to our cries?
> Can you ignore the appeals
> of the creatures your Son embraced?
> Can you refuse the prayer
> of Mary, his mother?
>
> Let us know the freedom of your kingdom
> where you live with your Son
> and with the Holy Spirit,
> one infinite freedom,
> for ever and ever. Amen.[4]

Mary, mother of Jesus, my mother, thank you for being a mother to me, for praying for me, for praying with me now.

Jesus, I come to you with your mother, the mother in heaven whom you have given to me. She prays now with me and for me. Amen.

Part III

JESUS, THE GIFTS OF THE SPIRIT AND INNER HEALING

SEVEN

&

Being Healed through Praise and the Gifts of the Spirit

THE FIRST WORDS of the prologue to Ignatius Loyola's *Spiritual Exercises* are: "Man was created to praise." This echoes Paul's Letter to the Ephesians 1:5-6: "*He destined us in love to be his sons through Jesus Christ, according to the purpose of his will, to the praise of his glorious grace which he has freely bestowed on us in his Beloved.*" Created to praise God as one of our most important activities, we can expect the Lord to make us more whole, more human, more integrated through doing something for which he made us: praising him. PRAISE HEALS. Rather, when we praise him, he heals us through our praise.

Praise

What do I mean by praise? For one thing, praise differs from thanksgiving. When I thank God, I show him gratitude for his gifts and, in my prayer, I refer those gifts back to him in my thanks. But when I praise God, I give him credit, so to speak, not for his gifts but simply for himself, "Praise is the point at which thanksgiving becomes thanking God for being God, or in the words of the *Gloria*, 'We give you thanks for your great glory'."[1] I can praise God for his actions, for the things he does, or I can praise him for his creation, or for any part of his creation; I can praise the Lord for anything and for everything, because he is the Lord of all things. Or I can just praise him for himself and for his qualities: his goodness, his love, his wisdom, his infinite greatness. I am not thanking him, precisely; rather, I praise him for being the kind of Lord he is, to have done these things, to have created these things to exist in this way, to act as he acts.

Praise is something like adoration, but more active, more going-out to God, speaking interiorly or out loud, or shouting, or singing, or dancing. Praise celebrates God. Adoration connotes the quiet or silent prostration of one's whole self before God (Rev 4:10; 7:11). Praise has voice:

> *"They cried 'Amen! Alleluia!' Then a voice came from the throne; it said: 'Praise our God, all you his servants, you who fear him, small and great.' Then I heard what seemed to be the voice of a great multitude, like the sound of mighty thunderpeals, crying, 'Alleluia! For the Lord our God the Almighty reigns'."*
>
> REV 19:4B-6

Praise gives nothing to God; it simply acclaims him, applauds him, for who he is. Praise acclaims the Lord now for what he has done, or does, or has always been and is. But praise does not look to the past nor even to the future; it looks straight at the Lord and claps its hands.

Praise means giving glory to God, glorifying him

through praise of his revealed glory. And so the First Vatican Council (1869-1870) declares that "the world was made for the glory of God"[2] This "glory of God" includes both the glory that God gives to his creatures and through which they manifest his greatness, and also the praise that we should give God as a response to the manifestations of his greatness. Nature and history show forth God's glory. "The world is charged with the grandeur of God; it will flame out like shining from shook foil" (G. M. Hopkins, *God's Grandeur*). And we are called to lift up praise to God, to glorify him in response to his glory that he reveals to us. Following Saint Paul, who writes that we are appointed and destined to live for the praise of the glory of the Lord (Eph 1:12, 14), Elizabeth of the Trinity wanted to be nothing other than "a praise of glory."[3] "Glory be to God," Hopkins writes, "praise him" *(Pied Beauty)*.

"Praise names," lists of laudatory titles recited to the king or to other illustrious personages, form the most important part of Bantu oral literature. Christian litanies are a kind of "praise names" to the Lord, and include prayer of supplication ("pray for us" or "free us, Lord" or "we beg you hear us" for example). The litany of the Holy Name of Jesus, the litanies of the Sacred Heart and of the Precious Blood of Jesus, and the litany of Loreto are good examples. The titles, the invocations — which vary, like "praise names"— are praise; the supplications, constant, complement them.

Many of the psalms are prayers or hymns of praise. They have a simple structure. A brief introduction sets the tone of praise: *"Praise the Lord! Praise the Lord, O my soul!"* (Ps 146); *"I will extol you, my God and King, and bless your name for ever and ever"* (Ps 145); *"Praise the, Lord all nations"* (Ps 117); *"Make a joyful noise to the Lord, all the lands!"* (Ps 100); *"Bless the Lord, O my soul"* (Ps 103 and 104). There follows the content of the praise, what the psalm praises God for: his creation (e.g., Ps 104 and 148); his goodness to us (e.g., Ps 103, 117 and 145); his mighty deeds (e.g., Ps 29 and 113). The conclusion repeats the opening shout of praise, such as "Praise the Lord," or *"O Lord, our Lord, how majestic is your name in all the earth"* (Ps 8), or sums up the main themes of praise in the body of the psalm: *"For the Lord is good, his steadfast love endures for ever, and his faithfulness to all generations"* (Ps 100).

Other psalms of praise are scattered throughout the Old Testament. These include Isaiah 25, which begins: *"O Lord, you are my God; I will exalt you; I will praise your name;"* Isaiah 42:10-13, *"Sing to the Lord a new song, his praise from the end of the earth!"*, and Nahum 1:2-8, which praises God for being *"a jealous God avenging"* (v.2). Moses' song of God's victory, *"I will sing to the Lord, for he has triumphed gloriously, the horse and his rider he has thrown into the sea"* (Ex 15:1-18), praises the Lord for saving his people from the Pharaoh's troops, for his power, and for his steadfast love. And praise is frequent in the historical books: Jehoshaphat appoints those who are to sing to the Lord and praise him in holy array, as they go before the army, saying: *"Give thanks to the Lord, for his steadfast love endures for ever"* (2 Chr 20:21).

In the New Testament, Luke's gospel and the Acts of the Apostles give an important place to praise. In the gospel, the praise begins with Mary's *Magnificat* (Lk 1:46-55), the song of Zechariah (Lk 1:68-79), and with the angels (Lk 2:13-14) and the shepherds (Lk 2:20) praising and glorifying God at the birth of Jesus. It continues with Simeon, who blesses God and praises him in a brief hymn (2:28-32) and the prophetess, Anna (2:38). Luke frequently shows those whom Jesus heals glorifying and praising God, as well as those who witness Jesus' healings and other miracles.[4] The blind man of Jericho, for example, his sight restored, glorifies God, *"and all the people, when they saw it, gave praise to God"* (18:43). In Acts: the Christian community (2:47), the blind man healed at the gate called Beautiful (3:8-9), converts (10:46; 13:48; 19:17) and all present (4:21; 11:18; 19:17; 21:20) praise and glorify God.

The letters of Paul often begin with praise, especially the letters to the Ephesians and the Colossians, and the two letters to Timothy contain bursts of praise. The Book of Revelation frequently refers to singing God's praises. The four living creatures sing, *"Holy, holy, holy is the Lord God Almighty"* (4:8); the twenty-four elders praise God, singing (4:10-11) and praying (11:16-17), and together they say *"Amen, Alleluia!"* (19:4).[5]

Christian worship has always emphasized praise, not only in hymns and in the divine office, but especially in the celebration of the Lord's supper; the Eucharistic liturgies, universally, are prayers of praise as well as of petition and thanksgiving.

Praise and Personal Integration

By praising the Lord, I open my heart to him. I take a stance of worship, going out to God on his own terms, not for what he does for me personally, but for who he is. And in opening myself to the Lord through praise, I open the door of my heart to his healing grace and to all his gifts; I become especially receptive to his Holy Spirit, who praises Jesus and the Father in me and through me, and in whom I offer praise to God.

Saint Augustine writes that praise does not help the Lord, adds nothing to him; but praise does aid us, serve us, help us to grow.[6] "Not that God grows through our praises, but that we do."[7] We grow in that, doing what we were created for and turning ourselves entirely to the Lord to whom we are headed, we become more ourselves,

more what the Lord has destined us to be from the beginning; that is, closer to him, more integrated as persons,
more healed.

The use, in praising God, of the gift of tongues provides
us with probably the best example of the Lord's use of our
own praise to heal us interiorly.[8] The gift of tongues has as
its purpose, prayer of petition, but also and predominantly, praise; it is chiefly a gift of praise. Studies have shown
that speaking in tongues, ordinarily at least, does not have
the structure of a real language. It goes beyond words,
beyond language. Praying in tongues is non-conceptual
vocal prayer, somewhat analogous to just being silently
and without concepts before the Lord. The principal use
of the gift of tongues is for personal prayer, although a
communal use is often found in prayer groups that praise
God together speaking or singing in tongues. When Paul
writes to the Corinthians to limit the use of the gift of
tongues in their prayer assemblies, he refers to *prophesying*
in tongues, a different use of the gift from praying in
tongues (1 Cor 14:28). Because of the very non-conceptual
nature of speaking in tongues, if used in prophecy in a
group, an inspired interpretation should follow; and again
because of its non-conceptual nature, tongue-speaking's
main function is quietly praising the Lord in personal
prayer. So Paul tells the Corinthians that, if there is no one
present to interpret prophecies in tongues, then let each
"keep silent in church and speak to himself and to God" (1 Cor
14:28).

Praise tends to shift and change the use of words.
Language breaks down under praise's weight. The aim of
praise is not to communicate messages, so the language of
praise usually omits the verbs and strings out titles in suc-
cession — "Lamb of God, Lord God, God Almighty"—
like Bantu praise names, like litanies. Praise tends to manifest an attitude, a way of beholding the one praised,

rather than to communicate precise meanings. And concepts, often, cannot hold the content of praise; words fail. Where praise transcends concepts, the gift of tongues begins. According to Saint Paul, praying in tongues builds up the one who prays, even though that person does not understand what he says in his prayer; because while his spirit prays, his understanding rests (1 Cor 14:14).

The gift of tongues is not a kind of ecstatic speech or utterance from a trance-like state, nor does it belong exclusively to any Christian group or groups. Peter Hocken has expressed it well:

Much misunderstanding and confusion stem from the focus on the language-aspect (any prayer of praise may not be linguistically impressive!) and from treating this phenomenon as "extraordinary". . . . From the nature of the case, anyone whose prayer has become predominantly the prayer of praise is near to praying in tongues; and it is really as simple as asking God for the extra push and letting it come . . . Of its nature [praying in tongues] requires a letting go of our self-control, of our tight grip on ourselves. It is within prayer a form of dying to self and rising to new life . . .[9]

One meets people who have no contact with Pentecostal churches nor with any kind of charismatic groups, but who have the gift of tongues and who use it in their personal prayer. It is not an unusual gift; on the contrary. The point should be made, however, that it is a gift, and that it is principally a gift of praise. The gift is not to make incomprehensible sounds, but that the sounds be prayer.

Sometimes the sentence of Saint Paul, *"We do not know how to pray as we ought, but the Spirit himself intercedes for us with sighs too deep for words"* (Rom 8:26), is applied to prayer in tongues. However, the Holy Spirit obviously does not take the place of the person praying. Rather, *the Spirit himself together with our spirit* (Rom 8:16) praises

God. Prayer in tongues is a rational act, even though under the influence of grace and having a non-conceptual content. It is "praying in the Spirit."

The content of prayer in tongues seems to come from unconscious or preconscious areas of the psyche, from regions of ourselves at the center of consciousness. Perhaps for this reason, praying in tongues has an intensely personal quality, expressing somehow the uniqueness of the person praying. Although not structured like other languages, praying in tongues contains the essence of language: not primarily the communication of ideas, but the expression to another (in this case to God) of the person speaking. Praying in tongues is a language the way that music, painting, and dancing are languages; it is praise as self-expression, the very self as praise, the beginning of the *new name which no one knows except the one who receives it* (Rev 2:17). Each gift of tongues is a personal and personalized language of prayer.

Again perhaps partly because the content of prayer in tongues seems to come from the below-consciousness levels of the one praying, the use of the gift has an integrating effect, heals the person praying — gradually over a long period of habitual use of the gift. In praying in tongues, the whole person — conscious and infraconscious, physical and emotional and spiritual, social and private — prays, and so a synthesis-in-action takes place, unifying all the strands and parts and fragments of the one who prays. The understanding, the intelligence, rests, subsumed into the whole of the person; western cultures tend to isolate intelligence and to cut it off from intuition so that it hardens into rigidity. In prayer in tongues, the understanding takes a vacation and gains new strength from the rest of the person. And the person gains a new spontaneity of expression and of existence. Praying in tongues unifies and integrates, and so heals interiorly, the person who uses it.

Morton T. Kelsey writes that,

> In many of the cases which have been
> observed tongues appears to be associated
> with growth and integration of personality. . . .
> Tongue speakers make it clear that there is an
> emotional release. One finds that it is easier to
> express emotions and to give way to them in a
> creative way. There is also a sense of joy even
> in the midst of difficulties. . . . Speaking with
> tongues is one evidence of the Spirit of God
> working in the unconscious and bringing one
> to a new wholeness, a new integration of the
> total psyche, a process which the Church has
> traditionally called sanctification.[10]

The Healing Gifts of the Spirit

All the gifts of the Spirit heal us in different ways. The Holy Spirit himself is the gift of Jesus and the Father, and his presence heals us.

The Father loves Jesus, and Jesus loves the Father; this mutual love between Jesus and the Father relates them to one another with a divine force that has its own personal identity. The relationship of mutual love between the Father and Jesus subsists as their Holy Spirit. The Father and Jesus relate us to themselves by sending us their Spirit; they catch us up into the life of the Trinity, into the divine community, by making us share in that which unites them in mutual love. In John's gospel, Jesus speaks of the Father and himself as "we": *"The Father and I are one"* (Jn 10:30); *"We are one"* (Jn 17:22). This "Divine We" extends to us: *"All should be one as you, Father, in me, and I in you; all should be one in us"* (Jn 17:21). *"If someone loves me he will keep my word and my Father will love him"* (Jn 14:23). Sharing in the divine "we" of Jesus and the Father through their Spirit in our hearts, we become more "we," more one, more united. The "Divine We" as such is the Holy Spirit who relates the Father and Jesus, and us to them and to one another.[11] The Holy Spirit is given to us by Jesus and the Father; he is Gift; and he is the Love who unites us to Jesus, to the Father, to each other, leading us to holiness.[12]

This means that every deepening of the relationship between Jesus and the person united to him involves a new sending of the Holy Spirit, a deepening of the Spirit's indwelling in that person's heart; we exist in a new way, closer to Jesus and to the Father in the Spirit. This new way of existing is what we call grace.[13]

The Holy Spirit manifests himself in our experience; we experience what he does in us. In Luke's gospel and in the Acts of the Apostles, the Spirit is the divine power. The angel says to Mary: *"The Holy Spirit will come upon you; the power of the Most High will overshadow you."* In this typical Hebrew parallelism, "Holy Spirit" and "power of the Most High" parallel and reinforce each other; they mean the same. The Holy Spirit is power. In the Acts of the Apostles, Jesus tells his apostles: *"You will receive power when the Holy Spirit comes upon you"* (Acts 1:8). In John's gospel, the Spirit, the Paraclete, comforts, consoles and strengthens us;[14] The Spirit *speaks* to us, shows us the meaning of God's word, and prompts us to witness to the words of Jesus.[15] In Paul's letters, the Holy Spirit *works* in us; he prays in us, he frees us (Rom 8:2, 26). He makes Jesus dwell in us (Rom 8:9-10; 2 Cor 3:18; Gal 2:20). He gives us the power to say "Jesus is Lord," and he manifests himself through his various gifts (1 Cor 12:3-4). All these operations of the Spirit in us speak of our experi-

encing the Holy Spirit. For this reason, the traditional for-
mulations of what the Holy Spirit does in us have been in
terms of experience. The Holy Spirit gives us his gifts:
wisdom, understanding, counsel, fortitude, piety, knowledge, fear of the Lord (see Is 11:2-3). We experience the
fruits of the Spirit in us: love, joy, peace, patience, kind-
ness, goodness, gentleness, self-control (Gal 5:22-23).

This list of what the Spirit does in all in whom he lives
do not of course define completely what he does in us;
they describe in an incomplete way the Spirit's activities
in every Christian. We can call these the common gifts of
the Spirit. Besides these gifts common to all to whom
Christ sends his Spirit, the Spirit gives special gifts,
charisms. Charisms are given to some, but not to all; however, the Body of Christ possesses all the charisms even
though no one member has them all. Saint Paul lists
charisms in various places in his writings, and of course,
none of these lists, nor even all of them taken together,
exhausts the variety and diversity of charisms that the
Spirit bestows. The classic list of charisms in 1 Corinthians
12, names as charisms: *the utterance of wisdom, the utterance
of knowledge, faith, gifts of healing, the working of miracles,
prophecy, discernment of spirits, and various kinds of tongues
and their interpretation* (1 Cor 12:8-10). In other places, Paul
also lists as charisms: teaching, helping, evangelizing,
administrating, leading, serving, exhorting, and alms-
giving.[16] The Second Vatican Council, in its Decree on the
Missions, names the missionary vocation as a charism.[17]
Evangelical poverty has long been understood as a
charism, especially since the great outpouring of poverty
in the early Middle Ages with Saint Francis of Assisi and
others. In the Jesuit tradition, the gift of tears has always
been considered a charism. And every religious order has
its own particular charism or clusters of charisms as
exemplified in its founders and in its greatest members.

A charism is both a call from God and the means to respond to that call. A particular charism enables a person to respond to the Holy Spirit in a special way, to receive the Spirit's action in a particular way. It makes the person a channel of the Holy Spirit in some special mode: according to leadership, or prayer, or mission, or healing, or government, or something else. A charism makes the Spirit "visible," as it were, or "tangible" in the Christian community. A charism is a gift for service, for the building up of the Body of Christ. But because the gift comes from God, a charism is primarily a new way of relating to God, a new way of being in Jesus.

Every charism, of course, is a gift; we have no right to any gift from the Lord. On the other hand, we do have the right and also the obligation to ask for the gifts that we need to be more healed. One has known missionaries who suffered from what can be described only as insufficiency of the charism of being a missionary. Those in positions of leadership can and should pray for new outpourings of the charism of leadership. Many persons who have answered the Lord's call to them to belong to him in a life of consecrated celibacy have prayed for an increase of the charism of consecrated celibacy (Mt 19:12; 1 Cor 7:7) and been healed in their emotions, in their total affectivity. There are, surely, special gifts of being a good Christian father, mother, husband, wife; where needed. And though these graces are given in the sacrament of Matrimony, the Holy Spirit can pour out charisms, special gifts, when we pray for them as needed. The Lord hears us when we cry out, and he answers. When we cry out for gifts that we need to be healed or equipped for his work, he gives them.

And sometimes the Lord does not wait for us to ask, but takes advantage of our openness to him in praising him, and gifts us with healing. Alleluia! "Praise the Lord"!

Lord Jesus, I praise you for you goodness to me.
And I ask you for a stronger gift of praise so that I
can praise you for who you are, for who you are for
me, and for what you do for me.

Praise to you, Lord, for the healing you give me,
especially for interior healing. Praise you because
you do all things well and at the right times and in
the right order.

I praise you, Jesus, for the gifts that you give me.
Increase your gifts in me so that I may be more
healed through your gifts and through using the
gifts that you give me, and so that I may serve you
better. Amen.

EIGHT

Jesus Is Lord

IN THE GOSPELS OF MARK, Matthew and Luke, the Kingdom occupies a central place in the teaching of Jesus; it is one of his main themes. In the Acts of the Apostles, and, especially, in the Pauline writings, the theme of the Kingdom becomes the theme of the Lordship of Jesus. This chapter describes the New Testament concept of Jesus' Lordship, then comments on the importance of this concept in prayer for inner healing, and finally reflects on the meaning of Jesus' Lordship for hope in the future.

The Lordship of Jesus in the New Testament

The key to the whole idea of Christ's Lordship is Jesus' use of Psalm 110.[1] This stands behind the early church's understanding that Jesus is Lord, and, surely somehow lies at the origin of the concept.[2] The application of the title "Lord" to Jesus occurs rarely in the synoptic gospels with the exception of Luke, who uses it eighteen times. It is not a title that Jesus applies to himself in his public ministry,

115

and — as Acts and the Pauline writings show clearly — the primitive Christian community understood Jesus to be constituted Lord by his passion, death, and resurrection. It is, then, to Jesus' use of Psalm 110 that one must look. The context is that of public exchange with the pharisees (Mt 22:41-46) and the scribes (Mk 12:35-37; Lk 20:41-44).

> *"Jesus, teaching in the temple, said, 'How can the*
> *scribes say that the Christ is the son of David?*
> *David himself, inspired by the Holy Spirit, stated,*
> *'The Lord said to my Lord, sit at my right hand till*
> *I put your enemies under your feet.' David himself*
> *calls him Lord, so how is he his son?' And the*
> *people heard him gladly."*
>
> MK 12:35-37

Psalm 110 is referred to again in the synoptic gospels in conjunction with a reference to the messianic passage of Daniel 7:14 (Mt 26:64; Mk 14:62; Lk 22:69), in the confrontation of Jesus and the high priest.

> *"Again the high priest asked him, 'Are you the*
> *Christ, the Son of the Blessed?' And Jesus said, 'I*
> *am; and you will see the Son of man seated at the*
> *right hand of Power, and coming with the clouds of*
> *heaven'."*
>
> MK 14:60-62

Jesus identifies himself with Daniel 7:14's son of man figure who comes with the clouds of heaven. But the phrase *"seated at the right hand of power"* is from Psalm 110: *"Sit at my right hand."* Here, having already entered into the paschal mystery, in his passion, Jesus identifies himself, by his use of Psalm 110, with the *"Lord"* to whom the Lord speaks in verse 1. The whole passion story itself, with a kind of sublime and mysterious irony that one can hardly grasp, speaks of Jesus as King and as Lord particularly in the passages concerning his being mocked, his conversation with Pilate, his presentation by Pilate to the people (*"ecce homo,"* and the inscription of the cross "King of the Jews").

How did the learned people of Jesus' time understand Psalm 110? Something can be gleaned from early Jewish literature on Psalm 110. Even though the Talmud and the Midrash were compiled much later than the time of Christ, they reflect opinions handed down from earlier periods. There is nothing in the Jerusalem Talmud, but the more important Babylonian Talmud contains two significant mentions of Psalm 110, identifying the (second) 'lord' with Abraham. However, the Midrash on Psalm 110, also equating Abraham and the 'lord,' points out that verse 1 of Psalm 110 is, at the same time, a messianic text. At any rate, Jesus' messianic use of the text tells us that it was considered, at least by some at that time, to be messianic. We can only speculate on Jesus' own study of Psalm 110 as "he grew in age and grace and wisdom," and of his use of it in his explanation of the scriptures to the two disciples on the road to Emmaus.

The early church's use of the title "Lord" for Jesus refers to the risen and glorified Jesus, with a certain emphasis on his divinity (he is at the right hand of the Father). The word "lord" *kyrios,* is the word for God in the Septuagint Greek of the Old Testament; in most English translations of the Old Testament, it is rendered as "Lord." Using the same title for Jesus, of course, is to say he is equal to God the Father.

Already part of the basic kerygma of the church in its first beginnings, Psalm 110 finds use in the Pentecost discourse of Peter (Acts 2:34-36), who concludes, *"Let all the house of Israel therefore know assuredly that God has made him both Lord and Christ, this Jesus whom you crucified."* Stephen, at his death by stoning, gazes upward and sees *the Son of man standing at the right hand of God* (Acts 7:56). And, further, some evidence shows that the mysterious "baptism in the name of Jesus" refers to the liturgical practice that had the person baptized say, during the rite, "Jesus is Lord."

In any case, the phrase "Jesus is Lord" is one of the oldest in the Pauline writings. It occurs six times (Phil 2:11; 1 Cor 8:6 and 12:3; 2 Cor 4:5; Rom 10:19; Col 2:6), and certainly antedates all the letters. Add to this the phrase, *marana tha* ("come, Lord") or *maran atha* ("the Lord is coming") of 1 Corinthians 16:22, a phrase which is repeated in the Book of Revelation (22:20b).

Perhaps most interesting is the passage of the Letter to the Philippians 2:5-11, which is so much commented on:

> "Have this mind among yourselves which is yours in Christ Jesus, who, though he was in the form of God, did not count equality with God a thing to be grasped, but emptied himself, taking the form of a servant, being born in the likeness of men. And being found in human form he humbled himself and became obedient unto death, even death on a cross. Therefore God has highly exalted him and bestowed on him the name above every other name, that at the name of Jesus every knee should bow, and every tongue confess that Jesus Christ is Lord, to the glory of God the Father."

"The name which is above every name" is the title "Lord," given to Jesus as the divine response to his suffering and death, to his "emptying out" of himself, his *keno-*

sis, which begins with his incarnation and reaches a high (or, rather, low) point in his death on a cross. The contrast between "the form of God" and "human form" is meant to be striking. The stress is on Jesus' humility and obedience ("even unto death") to the Father. In the final point of his *kenosis,* his death, Jesus descends into the heart of the world so that, in his resurrection, he can be the heart of the world, Lord in a true and even ontological way — not simply appointed or named juridically, but Lord in such a way that to uproot him would be to make the world cease to exist.

The same doctrine of Jesus' universal and organic (as opposed to merely juridical) Lordship is contained in the first three chapters of the Letter to the Ephesians. *He* [the Father] *has put all things under his* [Jesus'] *feet, and made him the ruler of everything, the head of the church — which is his body, and the fullness of him who fills the whole creation* (Eph 1:22).

The Letter to the Colossians (1:13-2:15), and especially what appears to be a previously existing hymn (1:15-20), views the whole universe as somehow suspended from Christ, anchored in him: *in him all things hold together* (v.17); *for in him all the fullness of God was pleased to dwell, and through him to reconcile to himself all things* (vv.19-20); the image differs from that of the Letter to the Ephesians, where Christ is seen as filling the universe. Here, in the Letter to the Colossians, the image is the opposite — of all things being (reconciled to God) in Christ; but the doctrine is the same: the universal Lordship of Jesus.

Because all creation comes under Jesus' Lordship, all of creation shares in God's plan of salvation.

> *"Creation still has the hope of being freed, like us, from its slavery to corruption, to have the same freedom and glory as the children of God. From the*

*beginning until now the entire creation, as we
know, has been groaning in one great act of giving
birth."*

ROM 8:21-22

The world is related to Christ through people in such a
way that the world itself is an object of salvation, of
redemption, of final transformation. Jesus, through us, is
the hope of the world and the guarantee to us of the mean-
ingfulness of the world. He is the Father's promise that
something permanent of what we make, suffer, work
through the world, will endure.

Furthermore, Jesus is the center of the Father's plan for
the world. God's plan, which has been revealed to us in
Jesus, is that all things on earth and in heaven be brought
together under Jesus as head, that all things be recapitu-
lated in Jesus. God has planned from the beginning of
time that all things that exist be reconciled, unified, har-
monized, in Jesus. This divine plan underlies human history and gives it its deepest meaning.

The Second Vatican Council, in "The Pastoral Constitution on the Church in the Modern World" *(Gaudium et
Spes)*, understands the whole world and all of history as
centered on the risen Lord. He is the goal of human history, the future focal point of all true progress. At its best
and most profound level, human history is moving
toward the ultimate reconciliation of all things in Jesus.[3]

Jesus is not only the goal of the world's movement into
the future; he is actively present in all of history and in the
whole universe. The fullness of the risen Jesus' active
presence and influence is in the church; but, at the same
time, his presence fills the whole creation (Eph 1:22-23),
which holds together in him (Col 1:17) in such a way that
everything depends on him and finds its meaning and its
value and even its existence in Jesus risen.

The Letter to the Hebrews (1:13) quotes Psalm 110 at the end of a series of proof texts to show the Lordship of Jesus (see also 8:1 and 10:12-13). And it goes further than the other Pauline writings in its use of Psalm 110, taking up the idea of the priesthood according to Melchisedek (Ps 110:4; Heb 6:20-7:20), thus associating Jesus' priesthood with his Lordship. The idea is that Jesus is not only Lord in his own right, but he sits at the Father's right hand as eternal high priest to intercede for us. He is our priest, our mediator, with the Father.

The Lordship of Jesus in Christian Life

Besides recognizing Jesus' Lordship over everything, we are called to recognize Jesus as our own personal Lord. Just as the Lord Jesus gives meaning and existence to the whole world, so he gives me my personal meaning and existence. Just as all history finds its true meaning and its fulfillment in Jesus, so I find my own true meaning and fulfillment in him. Jesus risen is present in all of history and in the whole universe, and he is actively present in my whole personal history and in every part of my life. I find my personal value, meaning, existence, and fulfillment in the risen Jesus.

Jesus has risen from the dead. His resurrection state of existence transcends all time, all space, all persons. Jesus risen is present simultaneously to every moment of time, past, and present and future. He stands present to every place in the universe, everywhere through his love. And the risen Jesus transcends all persons. This means that he is totally present to you now, as you read this. And he gives you his full attention. Now, and all your life, always.

What is more, Jesus loves you. Unconditionally, and without any qualifications. Your knowledge of him, in this life, has to be through love, a knowledge of the heart.

I can know Jesus through love. My own love for him is cold, small, inadequate. But I can know him mainly through *his* love for me. He loves me, and his love for me accepts me, forgives me, affirms me.

My knowing Jesus needs to be distinguished from knowing about him. I may not know much about Jesus, I may know no theology and be quite weak in bible study. But knowing Jesus is heart knowledge, not head knowledge. I know Jesus darkly, in the dark. Knowing Jesus through faith, through his love for me, can be — usually is — murky, dark, obscure, nebulous. I know him in a kind of cloud of unknowing. I know Jesus through love.

Just as the Father's plan from the beginning of time has been to recapitulate all things in Christ, to unify and reconcile everything in Jesus, so, too, the Father's plan is and always has been to unify and to reconcile everything in my being and in my life in Jesus, to integrate me, to give me personal unity, to knit up the frazzled parts of myself, in and through and under the Lordship of Jesus.

Jesus calls me not only to accept his love and his Lordship, but to participate actively in the Father's plan to recapitulate all things in himself. Jesus invites me to bring everything in my life under his Lordship: my worries, my problems, my anxieties and fears, my failures, my successes, my hopes for myself and for others, everything. I can take each preoccupation, every burden, all difficulties and sorrows and joys to Jesus, placing them in his hands, under his loving Lordship.

To the extent that I do, I will be co-operating with the Lord in his becoming the Lord of my whole life in a conscious way on my part. My prayer and my other activities will become more and more integrated so that my whole life becomes a prayer. My life will cease to be torn in two directions between an "upward" component of faith in

God, of worship and love of God, and a "forward" component of faith in other persons, in my work, in the whole human enterprise in general and in my particular part in that enterprise. I will stop being torn between the "upward" and the "forward." The Lord will heal me, make me whole, make an integration in me, a synthesis of all the elements and aspects of my life; he does this with my co-operation by which I bring everything in my life, consciously and explicitly, prayerfully, under his Lordship in conscious recognition of his Lordship over everything.

Distractions in prayer play an important role in Christian life. They show me where healing is needed in my life. A distraction such as a fly buzzing is minor, and when some person or project comes to mind, I can lift that person or situation briefly to the Lord. Rather it is preoccupations that are the real indicators: things that continue to come to mind; thoughts that disturb me. I can be praying and find my mind on another matter, on work to be done, on someone who is very ill, on someone who has hurt me, on a problem coming up. This kind of distraction indicates what is on my mind that is not integrated into my personal relationship with Jesus Christ. It shows up what is not under his Lordship, what I have not yet consciously and fully brought into the zone of the power of his love for me. If it is a distraction, falling outside my relationship with the Lord in prayer, then it is — in my life as a whole — not yet in his hands. In my prayer, I can put the matter into his hands, turning the distraction into a prayer. In this way, I co-operate with him in his work of reconciling the various things on my mind by bringing them into a unity in him; I let him integrate me, pull me together, become more the center of my life.

If I have a poor relationship with someone, I can put it in the Lord's hands, praying for that person and asking the Lord to heal the relationship and to fill it with his love and asking him to take the hurt out of it. If I am distracted by the thought of someone I love, or someone I am attracted to I can bring that person and that relationship to the Lord in my prayer, praying for the person and letting the Lord fill the relationship with his grace and his love, healing any selfishness or possessiveness in me and straightening out the relationship, guiding and strengthening me if the relationship is out of order. Distractions are clues as to what I should put prayerfully and explicitly under Jesus' Lordship for healing. Risen, he carries, glorified, the wounds of his passion, of his hurt. It is through those wounds I am healed.

My recognition of Jesus' Lordship is, itself, a gift: *No one can say "Jesus is Lord" except by the Holy Spirit.* (1 Cor 12:3). It is not so much that I claim him as my Lord, as that I let *him* claim *me.* I give up being lord of my own life, letting go and entering, with my whole life, freely and consciously into the realm of his Lordship by willingly accepting that Lordship.

To say *"Jesus is Lord"* is to celebrate Jesus' resurrection and his victory over the world, and to put one's whole self under his Lordship, allowing him to be my Lord.

Theological Reflection

How can we think of the Lordship of Jesus in such a way as to integrate into one meaning the two ideas that Jesus is my personal Lord, and Jesus is the universal Lord of everything? How has the *universal* Lordship of Jesus, a meaning on the *personal* level?

The Father's revealed word to us is, in the first instance, Jesus himself, risen and glorified. The totality of divine revelation is contained in the risen Jesus, and only in him. But Jesus, in his present glorified state, belongs — in some mysterious way — to the end of the world, as he who is to come. His resurrection happened as historical fact; but the resurrection event has one foot in history (the empty tomb) and one foot in the ages to come, in the New Jerusalem that Jesus inaugurates with his resurrection. That is, Jesus' own resurrection anticipates the final transformation at the end of history, and it somehow belongs, as the beginning, to that final transformation that marks the end-point of history.

We will not fully understand the Father's word to us in Jesus until history has reached its terminal point at Jesus' final coming. Although divine revelation is complete in Jesus risen, it will not be complete for us until history is over. This is true, also, because history itself reveals God and his plan; so revelation, as far as our understanding of it is concerned, will not be complete until history is completed.

Therefore, the full meaning of history will be revealed only at the end of time. The full meaning of anything, then, will not be seen until history's end. Further, the essence of anything is determined only by what it finally becomes. The essential identity of a person can be determined only by what that person ultimately becomes; this is part of the meaning of the parable of the workers who arrive at the eleventh hour (Mt 20:1-16) and of the conversion of the good thief on Calvary (Lk 23:40-43). Everything and every person is oriented toward its final consummation and fulfillment in the risen Jesus. Every creature finds its true meaning and direction in Jesus. This orientation of all things to Jesus is what we mean when we say Jesus is Lord.

The essence of anything, and the identity of any person is a function of that person's relation to Jesus — because he is the final judge who assigns to each its final post, its final meaning, and who will illuminate its entire existence utterly. So we are not yet what God has destined us to be from the beginning; we do not yet possess our true identities. Each of us is becoming, is in process toward our true self. We are becoming ourselves, and this becoming is a relationship with Jesus. In the Book of Revelation, the Lord tells us that at the end of this life, at the end of the personal history of each one, he will give to each person *a white stone, with a new name written on the stone which no one knows except the one who receives it* (2:17). This new name is the person's true identity, hidden now in the risen Jesus; and only then will I really be and know who I am. My authentic existence is in him, and the meaning of my life is hidden in him. So too is what I mean to him. The new and secret name will sum up how he sees me in love. It will be such a revelation of perfection, of completion, that it will keep me in a rapture of joy and love for eternity.

This is what is meant by creation in Christ. All creation, and every creature, is relative to Jesus, and finds its true self by going out of itself toward him, by leaving itself to find itself in Jesus Christ (Mt 10:39; Mk 8:35-36; Lk 9:24; Jn 12:25). God's creative act, that holds the world and each thing in it in existence, and that moves the world and each part forward (and this is history), is mediated through the risen Jesus. It is only in its relation to him that things exist (Jn 1:1-4; Col 1:16-17). And this mediation of the existence and the meaning and the fulfillment of everything is what we mean by the Lordship of Jesus. This is what we say when we say "Jesus is Lord."

We see here the relationship between hope and personal, prayerful relationship with Jesus. Jesus' resurrection, although a historical fact, belongs by its nature to the end of this world and to the world to come. It anticipates and inaugurates the next world. Furthermore, by reason of his risen state, Jesus transcends all space and time; he is present by his power and Lordship and active influence everywhere and always. Because he anticipates the ultimate future and all that leads to it, he contains that future — and the entire future — in an anticipatory way in himself. The future is, inchoatively, in Jesus. He holds the future in his hands, the future of the world and the personal future of everyone. For the Christian, Jesus Christ is the future.

And, present for me and holding my future in himself, he makes my future — hidden in him — present. In this way he is the ground of my hope. I can hope in the future because, even though I do not know what the future holds, I know who holds the future — Jesus Christ, who stands as the Father's promise to me of an ultimately successful outcome of my life, and who heals me of all fear of the future by filling me with hope in him.

Marana tha. Come, Lord Jesus.

Jesus, you are Lord. You are Lord of the whole universe; and you are my Lord, the Lord of my life. I take you now, once again, as Lord of my life; I profess you as my Lord.

I put my life under your lordship, into your hands. Each positive relationship in my life I put under your lordship. Each person that I hold dear, both the person and my relationship with that person, I place into your hands. Straighten out anything in that relationship that needs straightening or healing. Make any crooked ways straight, fill in any low points, level off any egoism or selfishness or possessiveness on my part in that relationship. Heal each one of these good and positive relationships in my life. Thank you, Lord.

Jesus, I put any and each negative relationship in my life under your lordship. Where you see in my heart resentment or anger or coldness toward the other person, put understanding and compassion. Where you see jealousy or envy, put gladness for the other person. Where you find in me fear of that other person, put courage and confidence and confidence in myself and the necessary assertiveness.

Lord, you are the lord of my future. I put all my future into your hands, under your lordship. I give over to you, Lord of my future, the rest of today, all of tomorrow, the rest of this week, what remains of this year, the rest of my life, and after my life on earth. I hand over to you each one of my worries about the future, for myself and those dear to me. I trust in you, Jesus, increase my trust, increase in my heart my hope in you. Amen.

NINE

❧

A Prayer for Inner Healing

JESUS SAID: *"When you give a banquet, invite the poor, the crippled, the lame and the blind"* (Lk 14:13). Jesus, of course, lives his own teaching, so we, who are interiorly poor, blind, crippled by hurts, qualify to be guests at his banquet. Our wounds shout after him. Is he willing to heal us? To the man who said tentatively, *"Sir, if you want to, you can cure me,"* Jesus replied emphatically, *"Of course I want to. Be cured!"* (Mt 8:3 JB).

One way of praying for inner healing is to take Jesus' hand and walk back with him through my life. He has always been there, loving me. He, in fact, thought me up, designed me from all eternity.

> *"Before I formed you in the womb,*
> *I knew you."*
>
> JER 1:5

> *"We are God's work of art, created in Christ."*
>
> EPH 2:10

Jesus knows my life in all its details. He remembers better than I do. And he has work to do for which he hopes to use me. Healed and free of the past, I can be more available, less crippled, more alive for him. *"I have come that they may have life, and have it to the full"* (Jn 10:10b).

So, Jesus, I ask you to go back with me to the time of my conception in my mother's womb,

> *"For it was you who formed my*
> *inward parts;*
> *you knit me together in my*
> *mother's womb,*
> *I praise you, for I am amazingly*
> *and wonderfully made."*

> PS 139:13-14

I can visualize my life as a staircase.[1] The time of my conception in my mother's womb is the bottom step. So, I stand on the bottom step and talk to the Lord about that time. My conception might have been a time of love and beauty, or a time of violence, distress and pain. The Lord knows. Perhaps I was conceived out of wedlock, or perhaps in violence. Maybe my mother was ill in some way when she conceived me. I put the fact and the time of my conception into his hands. I forgive anyone who might have hurt me in some way at the very beginning of my life. And I ask for Jesus' healing grace.

> *Lord Jesus, you were there when I first began to be.*
> *You called me into existence. Please heal anything*
> *in my conception, anything that remains inside me*
> *from the moments of my conception that needs*
> *healing. Come, Lord Jesus.*

My nine months in the womb were crucial for my subsequent life and attitudes. The dark dampness and warmth of my mother's womb may have been like a garden where I wandered with the Lord in the security of a prayerful, loving mother. Or it might have been a time of anxiety, sickness, economic deprivation, rejection. Whatever my mother and even my father went through in those months, affected me.

Perhaps I did not receive enough nourishment in the womb, or maybe I received nourishment that was not so good for me. There could have been some bad influences on my gradual formation inside my mother: smoking or drinking or psychological problems on her part, for example.

I talk to the Lord on this second step of my life, my months in my mother's womb. Again, I forgive anyone I might need to forgive, especially if I think I may have been an unwanted child, or perhaps threatened with a possible abortion or with an attempted abortion. These healings can go deep. I do not hurry. Stay with any phase for a long time if necessary. If persons concerned are still alive, some gesture of forgiveness may be helpful, however it might be received.

> *Jesus, you knitted me together in my mother's womb, you formed me. And you loved me then just as you love me now. Heal in me, Jesus, anything that you see needs healing that goes back to that time when you were forming me in the womb of my mother. Heal me, Jesus, and I will be healed.*

Jesus was there when I was born. I might have received rough handling from whoever helped me to be born, but I know:

"It was you who took me
from my mother's womb;
you soothed me on my
mother's breast.
From the womb I have
belonged to you,
and since the time that my mother
gave birth to me
you have been my God."

PS 22:9-10

Lord Jesus, you stood there by me at my birth. Take
that little baby that I was then, and that I am still
in some way deep inside myself, that newborn baby,
into your arms. Comfort me and console me. You
wanted me to be born, to live, and to grow. Heal me
now of the trauma of my birth, of the shock of
coming out of the dark and the warmth of my
mother and into the light and the noise and the
presence of other people. Jesus, heal the wounds and
the scars that I still carry deep inside myself from
the time of my birth and the time immediately
following my birth.

The next step on the staircase of my life is my child-hood years. I go through each year, remembering as far as possible, the people, the circumstances. I ask the Lord to go deeply into what I remember or have been told, of those years. Possibly I was hurt because my mother could not give me all the attention that I wanted. Or I could have been in competition for her attention, and for the attention of my father, with another child born before me or after I was born. Maybe we were poor, or suffered from the heat or the cold or from not getting enough to eat. I go back to those early years and try to remember as best I can how things were, how I was then.

> *Jesus, I thank you for my time at home, before I
> began school. I see in my imagination the place
> where I lived then, the various rooms, where I
> played, where I slept, where we ate. And I see you,
> Jesus, present in each one of those places, looking at
> me there, loving me, caring for me. Lord Jesus, I
> thank and praise you for my mother and my father,
> or for those who took their place in bringing me up.
> Thank you for the love present in my early life. I
> forgive my mother any hurts she might have caused
> me, wittingly or unwittingly, by her words or
> actions or attitudes toward me. I forgive my father
> for any failure to show me affection, to understand
> me; I forgive him for perhaps setting goals for me
> that I could not reach, for expecting too much from
> me.*

Then I move on to my early school years. The smallest
incidents are sometimes the most wounding, and they can
have a lasting influence. I may have been teased at school
for being too fat or too small, or for having the wrong
accent. I may have been unathletic or otherwise unaccept-
able to my peers. Worse still, there may have been bully-
ing, or unjust teachers against whom a child had no
redress.

> *Lord Jesus, you were there at the elementary school
> I went to. I remember the school as it was when I
> went there, the classrooms, the corridors, the
> lockers, the playground. And I see you, Jesus,
> present there, with me at school, looking at me with
> love, understanding me, taking my side when
> others may have been against me.*

I go now to the time of my pre-adolescence and adolescence, with the suffering I underwent during those years. Some of the hurts I suffered then, and that remain with me in some way now, have their origin in the sins of others against me. Some of the hurts are rooted in my own sins and sinfulness during the years of puberty and adolescence. I can pray:

> *Jesus, you grew up too. You have had your own pre-adolescence and your own adolescence. Heal the hurts that I received in my life during those years, painful for me in so many ways. My heart was broken during those years; Jesus, heal my heart. I suffered going through puberty; I did not understand the changes in my body and in my emotions. I did not know how to act; sometimes I felt like a fool, and sometimes I acted like one. I sinned. I know that you forgive me. Heal me. I suffered from my failures, in school and with others of my age. I found myself unable or unwilling to measure up to what other older people expected of me. I sinned against others and against myself. I failed often to take up my responsibilities. You are present Jesus in those difficult years of my life. Heal those hurts that are still, perhaps buried, with me and at the root of present problems in my life.*

In my adult life, right up to the present, I have been hurt. I want to invite the Lord into the memories of those hurts, not to take the memories away but to take out the hurt and pain and humiliation and fear and loneliness so that the meaning of what happened is changed.

> *Lord Jesus, in my adult life, I have been hurt. Please bring to my mind now the hurts that I have*

*undergone and the persons who have caused those
hurts. Show me the hurts that I should bring to
you, and the persons that you call me to forgive so
that you can heal the hurts that they caused. Help
me to see each of these persons in my imagination,
then in my imagination to put my arms around
that person and to say "I forgive you." And to see
you there, Jesus, putting your arms around both of
us and giving me the grace to forgive. Jesus, heal
my hurtful memories.*

As I move up the staircase of life, the type of hurts may
change. But often there is a pattern, a particular vulnera-
bility which others seem instinctively to seize on, so that
the same problem is repeated throughout life. A solution,
a breaking of the pattern, for example a pattern of being
always dominated by another, is to pray for forgiveness
for those persons concerned. I pray that the Lord forgive
them, and I pray for them, forgiving them from my heart.
This breaks the pattern, for I myself am bound if I bind
others. By setting them free, I am freed too.

> *"Forgive your neighbor the wrong
> he has done,
> and then your sins will be
> forgiven when you pray."*

SIR 28:2

Those whom we love can hurt us most. Jesus knows all
about this, *If anyone asks "What are these wounds on your
chest?" the answer will be, "The wounds I received in the house
of my friends"* (Zech 13:6). Yet not one word of reproach is
recorded when he met his friends after their desertion and
even denial of him, in his need. Furthermore, he chose to
keep the marks of his wounds, even the still gaping

wound on his side in his glorified body. *"Thomas, put your finger here; look, here are my hands. Give me your hand; put it into my side"* (Jn 20:27).

When I have finished praying for the healing of painful memories, I can pray for the healing of the roots of my sinfulness and for the healing of emotional problems. In particular, I want to ask the Lord to heal the roots of my habitual sins, especially the sins that undermine my human dignity and my self esteem, the sins that I hate myself for. These could be sins in the area of anger, impatience, impulsive outbursts against others, especially against those weaker than I am. They could be sins in the area of sexuality. They could be sins of failing to love enough those whom the Lord has put in my life for me to love. They could be almost anything.

I can ask Jesus to heal emotional problems. The Lord can answer prayer for the healing of depression, anxiety, fears of various kinds, feelings of guilt for sins that he has already forgiven, and other emotional and psychological problems. Jesus can heal these conditions wholly or partially through prayer, and he does. This does not mean that I should terminate any psychological or psychiatric treatment or therapy or counselling that I have been following. The Lord can and does work through medicine, counselling, and all kinds of therapy. But, also, I can pray; I can turn to him directly.

> *Jesus, I know that you love me. I am a sinner, and you forgive me completely in your unconditional and unqualified love for me personally. You love me not in spite of my sinfulness, but partly because of it. It is the opening in me for your compassion, that integral part of your great love for me. You came for sinners; you preferred to eat with prostitutes and traitors; you sought out sinful persons to make*

*them your followers. Heal the roots of my habitual
sin. Heal my ongoing sinfulness.*

*Lord Jesus, I hand over to you any emotional
problem that I have. I put myself completely into
your hands for healing any kind of depression, or
anxiety, or broken-heartedness. And I ask you for
healing.*

*Jesus, I give to you any guilt feelings for past sins
or crimes that I have already admitted and asked
forgiveness for. I know that you have forgiven me. I
accept your forgiveness, your compassionate and
merciful love for me. I forgive anyone who was
involved in past sins of mine, or who perhaps led
me into them. I do forgive them, and I ask you for
healing of the hurts that those sins caused in me.*

*Lord, I give you my fears. Please heal me of any
irrational fear, the fear of other people, fear of
persons of the opposite sex, fear of the dark, the fear
of animals.*

*Heal me, Jesus, of the fear of what other people
think of me. Heal me of the fear of failure.*

*Thank you, Jesus, for the healing power of your
love for me.*

I can pray alone for inner healing, or with a partner, or
with just a few people. I should choose them with care, as
being discreet, and very much attuned to the Lord. Any
advice or insights they may have, any suggestions as to
hurts being uncovered, should be discerned: *Do not quench
the Spirit . . . Test everything; retain what is good* (1 Thes 5:19-
20).

Notes

Chapter One

1. On healing in general: Francis McNutt, *Healing*, Notre Dame, Ave Maria, 1974 and *Power to Heal*, Notre Dame Ave Maria, 1977, and also *The Prayer That Heals: Praying for Healing in the Family*, Notre Dame, Ave Maria and Hodder and Stoughton, 1981; Barbara Shlemon, *Healing Prayer*, Notre Dame, Ave Maria, 1976; Barbara Shlemon Ryan, Dennis and Matthew Linn, *To Heal As Jesus Healed*, Resurrection Press, 1997; Matthew Linn, Sheila Linn, and Dennis Linn, *Simple Ways to Pray for Healing*, New York, Paulist, 1996; Jim McManus, *Healing in the Spirit*, Darton, Longman, and Todd, London, 1994; Benedict Heron, *Praying for Healing*, New Life, Luton, 1989; Michael Buckley, *His Healing Touch*, Collins Fount, 1987; Agnes Sanford, *The Healing Light*, Plainfield, NY: Logos, 1947; Morton Kelsey, *Healing and Christianity*, New York: Harper and London: SCM Press, 1973; Robert DeGrandis, *Layperson's Manual for The Healing Ministry*, privately published, 1985, Lowell, Massachusetts 01850.

2. On inner healing specifically, see especially: Matthew and Dennis Linn, *Healing of Memories: Prayer and Confession — Steps to Inner Healing*, New York: Paulist, 1974, and *Healing Life's Hurts*, New York: Paulist, 1978; Matthew Linn, Sheila Fabricant Linn, and Dennis Linn, *Healing the Eight Stages of Life*, New York, Paulist, 1988; Ruth Stapleton, *The Gift of Inner Healing*, Waco: Word 1976, and *The Experience of Inner Healing*, Waco: Word, 1977; Betty Tapscott and Robert DeGrandis, S.S.J., *Forgiveness and Inner Healing of Memories*, 1980; Michael Scanlon, *Inner Healing*, New York: Paulist, 1974; on inner healing as related to confession particularly, see Michael Scanlon, *The Power in Penance*, Notre Dame: Ave Maria, 1972.

Chapter Two

1. *Summa theologiae* I-II, q. 79, art. 4.
2. Ibid. I-II, q. 79, art. 3.

Chapter Three

1. See, for example, Claus Westermann, "The Role of the Lament in the Theology of the Old Testament" *Interpretation* 28, 1974, 20-38.

2. The translation is a slight adaptation of Delbert Hiller's translation in the Anchor Bible Series: *Lamentations:* New York: Doubleday, 1972, 96.

Chapter Four

1. For a theological reflection on Jesus' interior experience of his passion, see Gerald O'Collins, *The Calvary Christ,* London SCM Press and Philadelphia: Westminster Press, 1977. For a theological discussion of the meaning of the cross today, see R. Faricy, M. Flick and G. O'Collins, *The Cross Today,* New York: Paulist, 1978. For a spiritual theology of the cross in Jesus' life and in Christian life, see John Navone, *A Theology of Failure,* New York, Paulist, 1974.

2. Nor does anything else; a mystery is precisely something we can learn more about, but never fully understand *(Baltimore Catechism).*

3. Leopold Sabourin, in *Sin, Redemption, and Sacrifice,* Rome: Biblical Institute Press 1970, 167; Sabourin has an extensive study of reparation, 10-11289.

4. *The Prayers of Jesus in Their Contemporary Setting,* published by the Study Centre for Christian-Jewish Relations, London: 1977, 15-16.

5. This follows the careful and convincing exegesis of Ignace de la Potterie, in "La sete di Gesù morente e l'interpretazione giovannea della sua morte in croce," *La sapienza della croce oggi,* Turin: Elle Di Ci, 1976, vol. I, 33-49, who points out the need to read the phrase "I thirst" in the light of the other references of John's gospel to thirst.

6. J. Terence Forestell, *The Word of the Cross,* Rome: Biblical Institute Press 1974: "The primary symbolism of the water and the blood should probably be seen in the light of the same passage of Zechariah (13:1). In the context of the gospel, the water from the side of Christ can only symbolize the gift of living water which he promised to the Samaritan woman and of which he declared himself the source at the feast of Tabernacles. The death of Christ releases the streams of eternal life for men" (p. 89). Besides Zechariah 13:1, clean and purifying water that represents the Spirit of God in the New Covenant is referred to in Ezekiel 36:25; cf. Psalm 51:2; Isaiah 44:3.

7. Stanislaus Lyonnet, *Annotationes in priorem epistolam ad Corinthios* (class notes, Rome 1865-66), 44; quoted in S. Virgulin, "La croce come potenza di Dio in 1 Cor. 1:18-24," *La sapienza della croce oggi,* vol. I, 15.

8. Dennis Hamm, "To Heal as Jesus Healed?", unpublished paper written for and presented to an ecumenical conference, Roman Catholic and Assemblies of God, on divine healing. April 15-16, 1977, Springfield, Missouri, 4.

9. We have followed, with slight changes, John L. McKenzie's translation in the Anchor Bible: *Second Isaiah,* New York: Doubleday, 1968, 129-30.

Chapter Five

1. "Sermo de redemptionis nostrae" *Opera omnia,* vol. IX, Rome: Ad claras aquas 1901, 264c and 265d.

2. New York: Macmillan, 1969.

3. New York: Paulist, 1978, 239.

4. I, (Robert Faircy) am grateful to Matthew and Dennis Linn for the basic idea of this chapter and the previous chapter: that Jesus, in approaching his death, went through something like the five stages of dying of Elizabeth Kubler-Ross.

5. *The Cloud of Unknowing and the Book of Privy Counseling,* e.g. Image Books: New York, Doubleday, 1973.

6. See Matthew and Dennis Linn, *Healing Life's Hurts,* New York: Paulist 1978, 180-8.

7. Ibid., 236-7. The Linns also give valuable advice on how to pray for the healing of fear and anxiety about the future by meditating on Jesus' agony in the garden (237-8), and on praying to forgive as Jesus forgives by meditating on his seven last words from the cross (231-5).

8. The fourteen stations are: 1. Jesus is condemned to death; 2. Jesus receives the cross; 3. Jesus falls the first time; 4. Jesus meets his mother; 5. Simon of Cyrene takes the cross; 6. Veronica wipes the face of Jesus; 7. Jesus falls a second time; 8. The women of Jerusalem weep for Jesus; 9. Jesus falls a third time; 10. Jesus is stripped of his garments; 11. The crucifixion; 12. Jesus dies; 13. Jesus is taken down from the cross; 14. Jesus is buried.

For that matter, it is not necessary to stick to the number fourteen; in the beginning of the practice of the stations, from the early thirteenth century until the strong Franciscan preaching of the fourteen stations in the eighteenth century, we find anywhere from six to fifteen stations. For example the early seventeenth century Jesuits preached seven: Gethsemane, the house of Annas, the house of Caiaphas, Pilate's quarters, Herod's palace, Pilate's quarters a second time, Mount Calvary (see the *Dictionnaire de spiritualité*), vol. II, col. 2587); the seven stations have the advantage of being rigorously biblical.

9. *Le lettere di Santa Caterina da Siena,* ed. P. Misciattelli, Florence: Mazocco 1939, 36.

10. *The Revelations of Divine Love,* chapter 24; in the Penguin edition, 170; in James Walsh's translation, London: Burns and Oates, 1961, 87.

11. *The Spiritual Exercises of St. Ignatius,* trans. L. Puhl, Westminster, Md.; Newman, 1967.

12. Ibid., no. 53.

13. Ibid., no. 193.

14. Ibid., no. 203.

15. Ibid., no. 206

16. Ibid.

17. Ibid., 'Third Week' *passim.*

18. Stephen Sundborg, 'Ignatian Spirituality of the Cross' unpublished paper, 3.

19. Ibid.

20. *Exercises,* nos. 297 and 298.

Chapter Six

1. Leo XIII: Encyclical, *Jucunda semper*, September 8, 1894.

2. This prayer to Mary seems especially indicated where the hurts to be healed involve women — for example, a poor relationship with one's mother or sister or aunt, or a fear of women; also for the healing of resentment against authority.

This is traditional practice, to pray to Jesus for healing through the intercession of his mother. About the year 560, Romanos the Hymn Composer, as the antiphon verse of his hymn "The Leper," has this prayer for inner healing, to Jesus Christ: *Just as you cleansed the leper of his sickness, all-powerful One, by your mercy heal what is wrong with our souls, through the intervention on our behalf of the Mother of God, O you doctor of our souls....* (*Romanos le Mèlode hymnes*, Introduction, critical text, translation and notes by J. Grosdidier de Matons, vol. II, Sources chretiennes no. 100, Paris: Cerf, 1965, 360.

3. As does the eighth century Irish poet, Blathmac: *Come to me, loving Mary, that I may keen (lament) with you your very dear one.* What follows is a long poem of lament with Mary. Donal Flanigan, 'Mary in the Poems of Blathmac,' in *De cultu mariano saeculis VI-XI*, vol. III, Rome: Pontificia academis mariana internationalis 1972, 269.

4. Prayer from the English Missal, memorial of Our Lady of Ransom, September 24.

Chapter Seven

1. Peter Hocken, *You He Made Alive*, London: Darton, Longman and Todd, 1974, 79.

2. *Dogmatic Constitution on the Catholic Faith, Dei Filius*, canon 5 of chapter 1.

3. *Ecrits spirituels*, ed. R. P. Philipon, Paris: Seuil, 1974, 203-4.

4. Luke 5:25-26; 7:16; 13:13; 17:15-18; 18:43; 19:37-38; 23:47; 24:53.

5. See also 14:1-5; 15:3-4; 19:1-8.

6. Commentary on Psalm 102, *Corpus christianorum, series latina*, vol. 40, *Ennarrationes in psalmos CI-CL*, Turnholt: Brepols 1956, 1453.

7. Commentary on Psalm 134, ibid., 1937.

8. On the gift of tongues see: Robert Faricy and Lucy Rooney, *The Contemplative Way of Prayer*, Santa Barbara, Queenship, 1986, pp. 42-46.

9. Hocken, Op.cit., 83 and 82.

10. *Tongue Speaking*, London: Hodder and Stoughton, 1973, 220-2. Virginia Hine, looking at speaking in tongues, scientifically and in the light of other scientific studies, concludes: "Through a functional approach to the phenomenon, we have come to assess glossolalia [speaking in tongues] as a non-pathological linguistic behavior which functions in the context of the Pentecostal movement as one component in the generation of commitment. As such, it operates in social change...and in personal change, providing powerful motivation for attitudinal and behavioral changes in the direction of group ideals." *Journal for the Scientific Study of Religion* 7, 1969, 225.

11. H. Muhlen, "The Person of the Holy Spirit," in *The Holy Spirit and Power*, ed. K. McDonnell, New York: Doubleday, 1975, 27.

12. Thomas Aquinas, *Summa Theologiae*, III, q. 8, 1 ad 3; III *Sent.*, d. 13, q. 2, a. 2, sol. 2.

13. Thomas Aquinas, I *Sent.*, d. 15, q. 1, a..1 ad 1; d. 17, q. 1, a. 1; d. 30, q. 1, a. 3.

14. John 14:16; 14:26; 15:26; 16:7; cf. 1 John 2:1.

15. John 14:25-26; 16:12-23; 15:26-27. See H. Benjamin, "Pneuma in John and Paul," Biblical Theological Bulletin 5, 1975, 27-48.

16. 1 Cor. 12:28-30; 13:1-3; 14:6; 14:26; Rom. 12:6-8; Eph 4:11.

17. Section 23.

Chapter Eight

1. For a study of Jesus' Lordship in the New Testament, see: David M. Hay, *Glory at the Right Hand: Psalm 110 in Early Christianity*, SBL Monograph Series, Nashville, New York, 1973.

2. In the New Testament, Psalm 110 is most often referred to in terms of Jesus' sitting at the right hand of the Father, and so as an interpretation of the Resurrection and the Ascension. And it is used as a messianic text, frequently in conjunction with the word "Christ" (the anointed Messiah). So, although it is at the origin of the idea that Jesus is Lord, its use in the primitive church was chiefly functional, to explain what happened to Jesus as the Messiah in his Resurrection and Ascension: he was exalted, made Lord, given dominion, and sits at the right hand of the Father. However, it was used at the same time to express Jesus' Lordship, or dominion; it is sometimes used together with Psalm 8:6 (in Ephesians 1:21-22; 1 Corinthians 15:25, 27; Hebrews 2:6-8).

3. Number 10

Chapter Nine

1. The image of life as a staircase comes from Robert DeGrandis, *Layperson's Manual for the Healing Ministry*, privately published, 1985, available from HOM Books, 108 Aberdeen Street, Lowell, Massachusetts 01850.

Published by Resurrection Press

A Rachel Rosary Larry Kupferman	$4.50
Blessings All Around Dolores Leckey	$8.95
Catholic Is Wonderful Mitch Finley	$4.95
Christian Marriage John & Therese Boucher	$4.95
Come, Celebrate Jesus! Francis X. Gaeta	$4.95
From Holy Hour to Happy Hour Francis X. Gaeta	$7.95
Glory to Glory Francis Clare, SSND	$10.95
Healing through the Mass Robert DeGrandis, SSJ	$8.95
The Healing Rosary Mike D.	$5.95
Healing the Wounds of Emotional Abuse Nancy Benvenga	$6.95
Healing Your Grief Ruthann Williams, OP	$7.95
Heart Peace Adolfo Quezada	$9.95
Life, Love and Laughter Jim Vlaun	$7.95
Living Each Day by the Power of Faith Barbara Ryan	$8.95
The Joy of Being a Catechist Gloria Durka	$4.95
The Joy of Being a Eucharistic Minister Mitch Finley	$5.95
Transformed by Love Margaret Magdalen, CSMV	$5.95
RVC Liturgical Series: The Liturgy of the Hours	$3.95
The Lector's Ministry	$3.95
Behold the Man Judy Marley, SFO	$4.50
Lights in the Darkness Ave Clark, O.P.	$8.95
Loving Yourself for God's Sake Adolfo Quezada	$5.95
Mustard Seeds Matthew Kelly	$7.95
Practicing the Prayer of Presence van Kaam/Muto	$8.95
5-Minute Miracles Linda Schubert	$4.95
Season of New Beginnings Mitch Finley	$4.95
Season of Promises Mitch Finley	$4.95
Soup Pot Ethel Pochocki	$8.95
Stay with Us John Mullin, SJ	$3.95
Surprising Mary Mitch Finley	$7.95
Teaching as Eucharist	$5.95
What He Did for Love Francis X. Gaeta	$4.95
You Are My Beloved Mitch Finley	$10.95
Your Sacred Story Robert Lauder	$6.95

For a free catalog call 1-800-892-6657